Hatha Yoga Book 5

PRANAYAMA

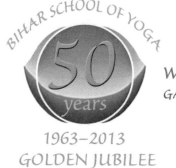

BIHAR SCHOOL OF YOGA

50 years

1963–2013
GOLDEN JUBILEE

WORLD YOGA CONVENTION 2013
GANGA DARSHAN, MUNGER, BIHAR, INDIA
23rd–27th October 2013

CONVERSATIONS ON THE SCIENCE OF YOGA

Hatha Yoga Book 5
PRANAYAMA

*From the teachings of
two great luminaries of the 20th century*

Sri Swami Sivananda Saraswati
Sri Swami Satyananda Saraswati

*Including answers from the satsangs of
Swami Niranjanananda Saraswati*

Yoga Publications Trust, Munger, Bihar, India

Published by Yoga Publications Trust
    First edition 2013

ISBN: 978-93-81620-75-5

Publisher and distributor: Yoga Publications Trust, Ganga Darshan, Munger, Bihar, India.

Website: www.biharyoga.net
         www.rikhiapeeth.net

Printed at Aegean Offset Printers, Greater Noida

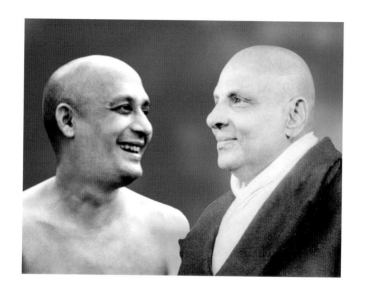

Dedication

In humility we offer this dedication to
Swami Sivananda Saraswati, who initiated
Swami Satyananda Saraswati into the secrets of yoga
and to our guru Sri Swami Satyananda Saraswati
who continues to inspire and guide us
on our spiritual journey.

Swami Niranjan

Contents

Preface

CONVERSATIONS ON THE SCIENCE OF YOGA

Conversations on the Science of Yoga is an encyclopaedic series which brings together the collected teachings of two generations of masters – Swami Sivananda Saraswati of Rishikesh and Swami Satyananda Saraswati of Munger. Satsangs given by Swami Niranjanananda Saraswati on his numerous national and international tours also provide the answers to many questions on this vast subject. These luminaries represent a living tradition in which the eternal knowledge and wisdom of yoga has been passed from guru to disciple in a dynamic continuum from the early twentieth century to the first decades of the twenty-first century.

The series consists of sets of books which present the timeless culture of yoga topic by topic, in question and answer format. In this way, complex and profound subjects such as karma yoga, hatha yoga and bhakti yoga, are presented in clear, simple language. These conversations on yoga reflect an ancient and enduring approach to the transmission of wisdom, in which spiritual aspirants seek answers to their questions at the feet of the guru.

Many of the answers also include verses from the various relevant scriptures, connecting the modern experience with the classical tradition. It is through the lives and teachings of the masters that the scriptures are correctly and intuitively interpreted for each generation, ensuring that the light of these revelations continues to illumine and inspire the hearts and minds of all who aspire for spiritual upliftment.

Conversations on the Science of Yoga has been compiled from the rich archive of satsangs and writings, both published and unpublished, which is held at the Bihar School of Yoga, Munger. The organization of this material into the major branches of yoga and related topics creates a unique interpretation of the classical yogic sciences for the benefit of humanity in the modern era. Deeply founded in tradition, the teachings are both systematic and practical, addressing the needs of individuals and society at a time when adjustment to constant change is placing unprecedented pressure on people all over the world.

The Bihar Yoga tradition
The Bihar School of Yoga is ideally placed to produce this major contribution to yogic literature. Founded in 1963 by Swami Satyananda Saraswati, the system known in India as Bihar Yoga and internationally as Satyananda Yoga, seamlessly integrates all facets of the yogic tradition, including the various branches of yoga, the philosophies which are fundamental to the yogic culture and the

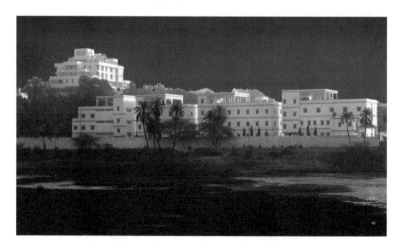

dynamism of self-realized preceptors which ensures that the teachings remain fresh and relevant in any age. This all-inclusive approach means that yogic practices are available as tools for holistic life management, while other *vidyas*, spiritual sciences, such as Tantra, Vedanta and Samkhya provide a broad philosophical base. Emerging from this living tradition, *Conversations on the Science of Yoga* is a unique and precious offering to humanity.

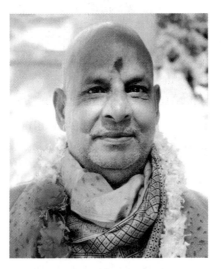

Swami Sivananda Saraswati (1887–1963)

Swami Sivananda was a towering spiritual force in the yogic renaissance which developed in India in the first half of the twentieth century. After serving as a doctor in Malaya, he returned to India to pursue his spiritual aspirations, and in 1924 was initiated into Dashnami sannyasa in Rishikesh. He founded the Divine Life Society, toured India extensively, wrote hundreds of books and inspired thousands around the world to practise yoga and lead a divine life. Swami Sivananda's eightfold path of yoga – serve, love, give, purify, do good, be good, meditate, realize – expresses his philosophy of service to humanity and continues to guide the work of the Bihar School of Yoga.

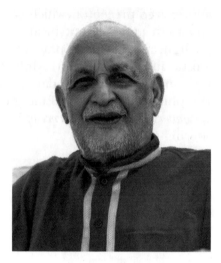

Swami Satyananda Saraswati (1923–2009)

Swami Satyananda was initiated into Dashnami sannyasa by his guru Swami Sivananda, in 1947. After serving his guru's mission in Rishikesh for twelve years, he founded the International Yoga Fellowship in 1956 and the Bihar School of Yoga in 1963. From that base he took the teachings to the rest of the world, fulfilling the mandate of his guru to 'spread yoga from door to door and shore to shore.'

Through his genius and compassion, many ancient, complex and esoteric practices were systematized, simplified and made available to people of all ages, cultures and creeds. Swami Satyananda's blend of charisma and pragmatism attracted multitudes of devotees wherever he went, giving rise to a global movement and creating a far-reaching network of ashrams, yoga centres and teachers. Meanwhile, the headquarters in Bihar continued to expand its many programs, including the publishing division, producing numerous books that both preserve and disseminate the incredibly rich seam of practical wisdom which flows through this lineage.

In 1988 Swami Satyananda renounced his mission in order to live as a paramahamsa sannyasin, performing higher spiritual and vedic sadhanas in an isolated location. During this chapter of his life, he also realized his guru's teaching of 'serve, love, give', by establishing Sivananda Math, an organization dedicated to raising the living standards of the weaker and underprivileged sectors of society.

At midnight on 5 December 2009, Sri Swami Satyananda Saraswati attained mahasamadhi.

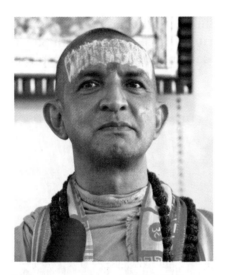

Swami Niranjanananda Saraswati (1960)

A yogi from earliest childhood, Swami Niranjanananda joined the Bihar School of Yoga in 1964 and was initiated into Dashnami sannyasa in 1971. At the age of eleven he was sent to live abroad by his guru Swami Satyananda, giving him direct experience and understanding of people from a vast array of cultures and walks of life. These years instilled in him a rare, cross-cultural insight into human nature, enabling him to communicate and interact with the international community with familiarity, ease and humour.

Combined with his depth of spiritual and yogic know-ledge, this background equipped Swami Niranjanananda to guide the Bihar School of Yoga and the international yoga movement from 1983 until 2008, when he began handing over the administration to the next generation. During this time he also authored many classic books on yoga, tantra and the upanishads and founded Bihar Yoga Bharati, the world's first yoga university, while continuing extensive national and international touring.

Following retirement from his role at the Bihar School of Yoga, Swami Niranjanananda established Sannyasa Peeth for the development and training of sannyasins, and for his own pursuit of the higher sadhanas of sannyasa.

As the spiritual successor to Swami Satyananda, Swami Niranjanananda continues to inspire aspirants around the world.

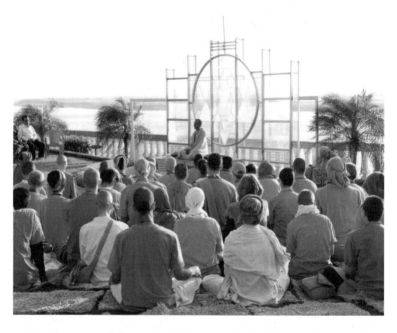

Yoga is not a philosophy, it is a practical science. Philosophy gives you knowledge, yoga gives you experience. This is the beauty of yoga. That experience is a manifestation of your inner being.

—*Swami Satyananda Saraswati*

Introduction

Pranayama is a method of refining the makeup of one's pranic body, one's physical body and also of one's mind. In this way, it is possible for a practitioner to become aware of new dimensions of existence.

—*Swami Satyananda*

Prana is the basis of life. Hatha yoga is a carefully constructed system of practices for the management of prana. Within hatha yoga, pranayama is the category of practice that is most directly involved with awakening, expanding and directing the pranas of the human body. Therefore, pranayama is a fundamental method for influencing one's experience of life.

What is this pranayama, which has so much power? And what is its medium for accessing the subtlety of the pranic body, which is invisible and unknown in common life? The answers, known in antiquity, have travelled through the abstraction of time to the reality of the present moment by two blessed vehicles: the scriptures, and the yoga gurus. In *Hatha Yoga Book 5: Pranayama*, the vidya of pranayama is thoroughly presented by those very means – the sacred books of India, and the gurus of a renowned sannyasa lineage.

Long before the medieval texts of hatha yoga recorded a codified and structured process for practising pranayama, the avataras and sages of the past revealed the purifying qualities of pranayama to their disciples. In *Yoga Vasishtha*, Sri

Rama is given pranayama sadhana for management of the mind; in the *Bhagavad Gita*, Sri Krishna instructs Arjuna; the *Yoga Sutras* of Sage Patanjali include pranayama as a limb of raja yoga; the Yoga Upanishads describe practices and their purpose. With the flowering of hatha yoga during the Middle Ages, books such as *Hatha Yoga Pradipika, Gheranda Samhita* and *Hatharatnavali* listed and described the pranayamas in more detail than ever before. Most recently, during the yogic renaissance of the twentieth century, master yogis of this era, Swamis Sivananda, Satyananda and Niranjanananda Saraswati, have further broadened the scope and application of this remarkable set of techniques, making knowledge of the power of breath and prana available for the benefit of all. *Hatha Yoga Book 5: Pranayama* brings together these multiple sources in a single volume, as questions from the basics of breathing to the highest application of pranayama in spiritual life are answered with reference to the scriptures.

Breath

From birth until death, the breath is one's constant companion. The ceaseless breath quietly continues as one goes about the vast array of activities and experiences that constitute life. Yet how many people are aware of the way they breathe? Unless there is a breathing crisis, few pause to consider the breath that sustains them night and day. Hence, few realize the influence their breath has on the way life is experienced.

In yoga it is said that the breath reflects the mind. Putting this knowledge to work, the yogis recognized that the mind can therefore reflect the breath – that is, by manipulating the breath, the mind is influenced. They also knew something else which deepened the implications of directing the breath: through the subtlety of their awareness, they recognized the breath as a vehicle for prana. Swami Sivananda expresses this understanding when he says, "Pranayama begins with the regulation of breath and ends in establishing full and perfect control over the life currents or vital inner forces."

Before learning the classical pranayamas, therefore, one must develop correct breathing and become adept at certain basic breathing methods. In Satyananda Yoga these are systematically outlined, and for many people, these practices alone transform both physical and mental health. The solution to debilitating conditions such as insomnia, indigestion, headache, chest pain, anxiety, panic and anger can be as simple as learning how to breathe fully. The breath is ever-present; with the knowledge of breath management one has constant access to a tool for strengthening the body and managing the mind. Swami Niranjan says, "Nothing is closer than one's own breath. It is tangible, believable, understandable and controllable. The gentle inhalation and exhalation is sustaining and calming, it affects one's thoughts and is itself affected by one's activities, emotions and thoughts."

Once the basic breathing techniques have been mastered, pranayamas can be gradually learned, and the sadhaka enters the realm of true hatha yoga. Until then, one is practising *prana nigraha*, control of the breath. This is an essential and transformative stage which must not be undervalued; for when the connection is made between breath and prana, it becomes clear that the profound effect of the breath on the mind is a principle theme of hatha yoga.

Purification

Hatha yoga talks much of purifying the *nadis*, the channels of prana in the body. Of the 72,000 nadis, hatha yoga is chiefly concerned with strengthening and balancing the two major flows, known as ida and pingala. Once this is achieved, the awakening of *sushumna*, the spiritual nadi, becomes possible. *Ida nadi* is the energy of the mind, while *pingala nadi* is the dynamic or physical energy. The pranayama practice of *nadi shodhana*, often referred to as alternate nostril breathing, is correctly translated as 'nadi purification'. Here, the connection between breath, pranayama and mind comes into focus, as it is seen how the manipulation of the breath in the left and right nostrils directly affects the mental energy and its relationship with the physical energy. Swami Satyananda beautifully describes the intimate relationship of breath and mind when he says, "The moment the mind becomes active, the breath is also resurrected, because the mind and the breath are two companions. They live together, move together, fly together and die together."

Modern science has added a further dimension to the understanding of nadi shodhana's remarkable ability to integrate the personality and remove inner conflict. Knowledge of the 'split' brain, meaning the different functions of the left and right brain hemispheres, shows correlations with the characteristics of ida and pingala nadis. Ida and pingala are associated with the flows of breath in the left and right nostrils, and it is now known that the flow of breath in each nostril activates the opposite brain hemisphere. With this discovery, a scientific explanation validates the power of the ancient system of pranayama, taking hatha yoga into a new era. Research into the mechanisms behind yoga practices has been a key contribution of Bihar School of Yoga to the development of yoga today. This aspect is also explored in *Pranayama*, as science and pranayama, and the effects of pranayama on the brain are discussed in detail.

Sadhana and lifestyle

In Satyananda Yoga classes and daily sadhana, pranayama is included as a component of the overall session: it follows asanas and prepares one for meditation. In this way its benefits are optimized and an integrated sadhana of hatha and raja yoga is made cohesive, with pranayama becoming the bridge from hatha yoga to raja yoga.

The traditional texts talk of pranayama sadhana as a sadhana in its own right, describing an intensity of practice which is not advisable for the average householder. Such sadhanas require a rigorous and disciplined lifestyle and practice routine under the direct guidance of a guru.

4

Nevertheless, the instructions given for such practice can guide the general student towards healthy living, always bearing in mind the practicalities of one's individual situation. These guidelines include diet, place of living, level of association with others, time and regularity of practice. The wisdom of the sages explains that without an appropriate lifestyle and attitude, the fruits of pranayama will be limited. Therefore, it should not be expected that half an hour of practising yoga each day can compensate for an indulgent and unbalanced lifestyle. Establishing a simple, harmonized way of life is regarded as part of spiritual living and is essential preparation for advancing in yogic sadhana.

Categories of pranayama

Once the foundation of breath correction, basic breathing methods, simple nadi shodhana and lifestyle are in place, pranayama and its applications can be explored in more depth. Satyananda Yoga has categorized the pranayama practices into several groupings, based on their characteristics and effects. These categories help practitioners to apply the techniques appropriately, which is the aim of pranayama in the modern context. This is an important point which applies not only to pranayama, but to the whole range of practices made available by the gurus of these times.

Nadi shodhana is the major balancing pranayama, consisting of many stages, taking one from the simplest to a most advanced sadhana which few will accomplish. In *Pranayama*, the discussion on nadi shodhana is extensive, reflecting its significance both as a traditional sadhana and its importance for helping bring harmony into everyday life.

The tranquillizing pranayamas have a particularly calming effect on the body-mind, quickly activating the parasympathetic nervous system, or relaxation response. They are, therefore, the ideal tool for stress minimization. By regular practice, the relaxation response becomes stronger and therefore more accessible at times of stress.

5

This also enables faster recovery from stress. Such practices are extremely effective at relieving anxiety and any delayed effects of trauma.

The vitalizing pranayamas are energizing and as such raise the level of vitality and health when practised regularly. They are helpful in lifting the mood and are used in programs to shift depression and fatigue. It needs to be remembered that they are powerful techniques, however, and must be used with care: the contra-indications should always be observed, and practice needs to be moderate, as guided by an experienced teacher.

Advanced pranayama involves incorporation of breath retention and other yogic techniques of mudra and bandha. Such practices are for those adopting yoga as a method for spiritual evolvement. They take one into the realm of pranayama as a sadhana in spiritual life, the final chapter of *Pranayama*. Here, the role of pranayama in meditation, kundalini awakening and the attainment of *samadhi*, the highest state of sublime consciousness, is revealed by those who have walked the path and know the way.

Swami Niranjan sums up the brilliance of pranayama when he says, "Although the practices have innumerable physical benefits, the therapeutic aspect of pranayama is an incidental by-product. The practitioner of pranayama will certainly experience many benefits at the physical level. These effects have been documented scientifically, and it has been observed that pranayama influences almost all the organs and physiological systems. The main objective of pranayama, however, is to balance the interacting processes of the pranic and mental forces for awakening the higher centres of human consciousness: the real purpose of pranayama is to awaken the pranas, chakras and kundalini."

Note

Hatha Yoga Book 5: Pranayama is not an instruction book. Pranayama should always be learned from a qualified teacher with understanding of contra-indications and precautions.

1

Understanding Pranayama

PRANA

What is prana?

Swami Sivananda: Prana is the link between the physical and the astral bodies. When the slender, thread-like prana is cut off, the astral body separates from the physical body. Death is the result. The prana that was working in the physical body is withdrawn into the astral body.

Prana digests the food, turns it into chyle and blood, and sends it into the brain and the mind. The mind is then able to think and reflect on the self in meditation.

Prana is the universal principle of energy or force. It is vital force. Prana is all-pervading. It may be either in a static or dynamic state. It is found in all forms, from the lowest to the highest, from the ant to the elephant, from the unicellular amoeba to a man, from the elementary form of plant life to the developed form of animal life.

It is prana that shines in your eyes. It is through the power of prana that the ear hears, the eye sees, the skin feels, the tongue tastes, the nose smells, the brain and the intellect perform their respective functions. The smile on the face of a young lady, the melody in music, the power in the emphatic utterances of an orator, the charm in the words of one's own beloved wife – all these and many more have their origin in prana. Fire burns through prana. Wind blows through prana.

Rivers flow through prana. The steamer and the airplane, the train and the motor car move about only through the power of prana. Radio waves travel through prana. Prana is electron. Prana is proton. Prana is force. Prana is magnetism. Prana is electricity. It is prana that pumps blood from the heart into the arteries. It is prana again that does digestion, excretion and secretion.

Prana is expended by thinking, willing, acting, moving, talking, writing and so on. A strong and healthy man has an abundance of prana or vitality. The prana is supplied by food, water, air and solar energy. The supply of prana is received by the nervous system. The prana is absorbed in breathing. The excess of prana is stored up in the brain and nerve centres. When the seminal energy is sublimated, it supplies an abundance of prana to the system.

How important is prana in the functioning of the body?

Swami Niranjanananda: In *Prashnopanishad* there is a discussion on the subject of prana. It says that prana is the lord of all the expressions of the human body. A story is told.

Once upon a time, there was a conflict between the energies, forces, faculties and senses or *devas* that reside in the body. Each one said, "I am the important one, without me you would not be able to function". Buddhi said, "Without me you wouldn't be able to discriminate." The eyes said, "Without us you wouldn't be able to recognize anything." The legs said, "Without us you would not be able to move." The hands said, "We are the important ones", and there was great confusion. Prana was listening quietly; fed up with all the bickering and fighting, he decided to retire. Unfortunately, when he retired everything died. He had to be called back again and the other forces recognized him as their lord.

In *Prashnopanishad* (2:4) it is thus written:

Sobhimaanaat oordhvam utkramata iva
tasminnutkraamatyathetare sarva evotkraamante
tasminschcha pratishthamaane sarva eva praatishthante;
Tadyathaa makshikaa madhukararaajaanam utkraamantam
sarvaa makshikaa madhukararaajaanam utkraamantam
sarvaa evotkraamante tasminshcha pratishthamaane sarvaa
eva praatishthanta evam vaanmanashchakshuh shrotram cha
te preetaah pranam stunvanti.

In a fit of wrath, prana withdrew himself from the body. Immediately, all the deities found themselves leaving with him, and when prana returned the deities found themselves back in their former places. Just as bees leave the hive when their queen departs and return when she returns, so did the deities behave. Satisfied with this evidence, the deities now give worship to prana.

This prana is in our material body, the physical dimension, in five different forms known as the *pancha pranas* or five pranas. They are: prana, apana, samana, udana and vyana. It is a subtle activity taking a physical form. The physical manifestation of prana, apana, samana, udana or vyana cannot be seen, yet their manifestation outwards is through the body.

What is the relationship between prana and pranayama?

Swami Niranjanananda: In *Yoga Vasishtha* Sri Rama asks his guru Sage Vasishtha a question: "You are telling me many things, but are there any practical ways in which I can experience them?" Sage Vasishtha answers, "Yes, O Rama, practise pranayama." Why does Sage Vasishtha suggest the practice of pranayama?

According to the yogic concepts, there are three flows in the body: the solar force, the lunar force, and the balanced force. The solar force is known as *pingala*, the lunar force is known as *ida* and the balanced force is known as *sushumna*. The three flows are carriers of a specific gross, subtle and spiritual energy.

Pingala is the gross energy, *prana shakti*. The body functions because of prana shakti. In the absence of prana, one is devoid of physical life. Ida is the *chitta shakti*, the mental force. The mind is sustained and nurtured by this flow of ida shakti, the subtle prana. The spiritual nature of every individual is nurtured by sushumna, the balance of both. Sage Vasishtha tells Sri Rama, "If the body is disturbed, or if it is experiencing ill health, you can manage all the imbalances and rectify all the defects and diseases of your body by awakening prana shakti."

This has been seen in the life of yogis who are able to manage many physical conditions with the practice of pranayama. Even asana is not necessary, as pranayama increases the vital energy, the prana shakti, and removes the blocks of prana.

Disease occurs when there is a block of prana. Headache occurs when there is a block of prana. Eyesight is lost when there is a block of prana in the eyes, hearing is lost when there is a block of prana in the ears, and speech is lost when there is a block of prana at the throat in the speech centre. Digestion becomes sluggish when there is a loss of prana in the digestive system. Muscles become weak when there is a loss of prana in the muscular system. Nervous tensions and nervousness arise when there is a loss of prana in the nervous system. Respiratory problems occur when there is a loss of prana in the respiratory organs. In *Prashnopanishad* (2:12) it is written:

Yaa te tanoorvaachi pratishthitaa yaa cha chakshushi;
Yaa cha manasi santataa shivam taam kuru motkrameeh.

O prana, remain in the body calm and quiet; do not leave the body. You are the Lord who abides within the speech, ear, eye and mind.

That is the theory and concept of yoga therapy. Remove the blocks to prana which are afflicting a particular organ or system or location within the body. Many yogis practise pranayama as their sadhana. They have no blocks in their body; they are in optimum health.

In the same manner, once the mental prana, the chitta shakti, also becomes active and powerful all the activities of the mind can be controlled, guided and calmed. Therefore, Sage Vasishtha talks of pranayama practice to Sri Rama and tells him, "Pranayama is a method by which you can regulate the functions and the deficiencies of your body and mind."

What is the power of prana?

Swami Niranjanananda: In 1977 Sir Edmund Hilary, the man who conquered Mount Everest, made a trip. He followed the path of the river Ganga, from Ganga Sagar, the place where Ganga merges into the ocean, to the source of Ganga in the Himalayas. He went up the river, travelling in three powerful rocket boats to go against the current of the river. When he was travelling along the meandering river above the Rishikesh area, he saw an emaciated yogi in the middle of the river, seated on a rock. Sir Edmund stopped near the rock and called out to the yogi seated there, "What are you doing?" The yogi said, "I am practising pranayama." Hillary said, "What is the attainment of pranayama?" The yogi said, "Nothing, only vitality." They had a chat for about ten minutes.

Then Sir Edmund decided to continue on his journey. While he was talking to the yogi the three boats had anchored. They had tied the rope to the rock as an anchor. The ropes were unhitched, the engines started and the boats put in forward gear. However, the boats did not move. The engines were checked, everything was fine: the rev was fine, there was power and fuel, so what was wrong? At that moment Sir Edmund happened to look back and saw the emaciated yogi seated on that rock in the middle of the Ganga holding the three ropes in his hand. He was holding back the boats.

This story was published in the *Times of India* in 1977. It is an indication of the power of prana shakti in a yogi whose

11

body is just skin and bones. He was holding the ropes of three powerful motor boats and all the revs of the engines could not move them forward. Therefore, do not think of prana as breath, but as the force of life.

What are the pancha koshas?
Swami Niranjananananda: According to yoga, a human being is capable of experiencing five dimensions of existence, which are called *pancha kosha*, or five sheaths. These are the five spheres in which a human being lives at any given moment and they range from gross to subtle. The pancha koshas are: i) annamaya kosha, ii) pranamaya kosha, iii) manomaya kosha, iv) vijnanamaya kosha and v) anandamaya kosha.

The first sheath or level of experience is the physical body, or *annamaya kosha*. The word *anna* means, food and *maya* means, comprised of. This is the gross level of existence and is referred to as the food sheath due to its dependence on food, water and air. This sheath is also dependent on prana.

The second sheath is *pranamaya kosha*, the energy field of an individual. The level of experience here is more subtle than the physical body, which it pervades and supports. This sheath is supported in turn by the subtler koshas. Together, the physical and pranic bodies constitute the basic human structure, which is referred to as *atmapuri*, the city of the soul. They form the vessel for the experience of the higher bodies.

The pranamaya kosha is the basis for the practices of pranayama and prana vidya. It is also described as the pranic, astral and etheric counterpart of the physical body. It has almost the same shape and dimensions as its flesh and blood vehicle, although it is capable of expansion and contraction. It has been said in the *Tattiriya Upanishad* (*Brahmandavalli*: 2a):

Tasmaadvaa etasmaadannarasamayaado'ntara aatmaa praanamayah;
Tenaisha poornah.

Sa vaa esha purushavidha eva;
Tasya purushavidhataamanvayam purushavidhah.

Verily, besides this physical body, which is made of the essence of the food, there is another, inner self comprised of vital energy by which this physical self is filled. Just as the fleshly body is in the form a person, accordingly this vital self is in the shape of a person.

Clairvoyants see the pranic body as a coloured, luminous cloud or aura around the body, radiating from within the physical body like the sun flaring from behind the eclipsing moon.

The third sheath is *manomaya kosha*, the mental dimension. The level of experience is the conscious mind, which holds the two grosser koshas, annamaya and pranamaya, together as an integrated whole. It is the bridge between the outer and inner worlds, conveying the experiences and sensations of the external world to the intuitive body, and the influences of the causal and intuitive bodies to the gross body.

The fourth sheath is *vijnanamaya kosha*, the psychic level of experience, which relates to the subconscious and

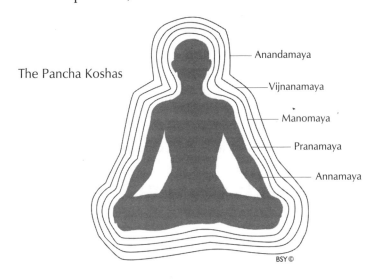

The Pancha Koshas

Anandamaya

Vijnanamaya

Manomaya

Pranamaya

Annamaya

BSY©

13

unconscious mind. This sphere pervades manomaya kosha, but is subtler than it. Vijnanamaya kosha is the link between the individual and the universal mind. Inner knowledge comes to the conscious mind from this level. When this sheath is awakened, one begins to experience life at an intuitive level, to see the underlying reality behind outer appearances. This leads to wisdom.

The fifth sheath is *anandamaya kosha*, the level of bliss and beatitude. This is the causal or transcendental body, the abode of the most subtle prana.

What is the role of prana in the five koshas?

Swami Niranjanananda: All the five sheaths are pervaded by prana, which nourishes and sustains them, and maintains their appropriate relationship. The movement from one kosha to another is also achieved with the help of prana. How prana operates in between the koshas can be understood by the example of a gearshift in a car. One moves in between the gears through the neutral. Neutral is not a gear – the gears are first, second, third, fourth and reverse. Without the neutral space in between, however, one cannot shift from one gear to another. The same principle applies to the koshas.

The pranamaya kosha acts as the neutral space, allowing one to move from annamaya to manomaya, manomaya to vijnanamaya, vijnanamaya to anandamaya, and so on. One must use the faculty of prana shakti in order to move from any one state to another. With the activation of prana, one gains access to the physical, mental, psychic and spiritual dimensions.

How is the pranamaya kosha affected by lifestyle?

Swami Satyananda: Lifestyle has a profound impact on the pranamaya kosha and its pranas. Physical activities such as exercise, work, sleep, intake of food and sexual relations all affect the distribution and flow of prana in the body. Faculties of the mind such as emotion, thought and imagination affect the pranic body even more.

Irregularities in lifestyle, dietary indiscretions and stress deplete and obstruct the pranic flow. This results in what people experience as being 'drained of energy'. Depletion of energy in a particular prana leads to the devitalization of the organs and limbs it governs and ultimately to disease or metabolic dysfunction. The techniques of pranayama reverse this process, energizing and balancing the different pranas within pranamaya kosha. In an integrated yoga program pranayama practices should be performed after asanas.

How can the power of pranayama be understood?

Swami Satyananda: *Pranayama* is the science of the universal energy, of universal mind, of universal time, space and matter. That is the complete meaning of pranayama. The practice of pranayama has a direct link, a direct effect on the most intricate and sophisticated functioning of the brain. It is not the air one breathes that constitutes pranayama, it is the vital, universal pranic energy which is present in all people, and which has to be dynamized and redistributed. That is the science of pranayama.

WHAT IS PRANAYAMA?

What is to be attained by practising pranayama?

Swami Sivananda: Start the practice of pranayama this very second in right earnest! Control the breath and calm the mind. Steady the breath and enter samadhi. Restrain the breath and lengthen the life. Subdue the breath and become a yogi – a dynamo of power, peace, bliss and happiness.

What does the process of pranayama involve?

Swami Sivananda: Pranayama means the control of prana and the vital forces of the body. Pranayama begins with the regulation of breath and ends in establishing full and perfect control over the life currents or vital inner forces. In other words, pranayama is the perfect control of the life currents through regulation of the breath. Breath is the external

15

manifestation of the gross prana. By establishing control over the gross prana, control can easily be gained over the subtle prana inside. The process by which such control is established is called pranayama.

What is the real meaning of pranayama?

Swami Satyananda: Pranayama is a greatly misunderstood term. People translate it as 'breathing exercise'. Of course the practices do improve the introduction of oxygen into the physical body and the removal of carbon dioxide. Of this there is no doubt, and this in itself brings about wonderful physiological benefits. But pranayama is not simply a respiratory exercise, or an exercise of the breath. Pranayama does not mean controlling the life force. Pranayama does not mean controlling the breath. Then what is pranayama? Pranayama means conveying the life force to every nook and corner of the body.

It is actually a process which awakens the dormant prana, the sleeping vital energy in the physical body. It is part of a total system of reintegration, rebalancing and reharmonizing of body and mind, a system which purifies and strengthens, and thereby eliminates physical and mental tension and weakness. Simultaneously, pranayama awakens the inner awareness.

The practice of pranayama recharges the energy in the physical body which is then conducted by ida and pingala nadis in the form of electrical impulses to all parts of the body, including the brain. Scientists have observed that when pranayama is practised both hemispheres of the brain are active and there are great changes in the brain's electrical impulses.

What is the meaning and significance of the word pranayama?

Swami Satyananda: Prana, means far more than breath. 'Prana' plus 'ayama' gives 'prana-ayama'. *Ayama* is a Sanskrit word which can be defined as follows: stretching, extending, restraining, expansion (of dimensions in time and space).

Thus, pranayama means to extend and overcome one's normal limitations. Pranayama uses the breathing process as a means to manipulate all forms of prana within the human framework, whether gross or subtle, but it is chiefly concerned with influencing the subtle forms of prana. Pranayama provides the method whereby one is able to attain higher states of vibratory energy. In other words, one is able to activate and regulate the prana within the human framework and thereby make oneself more sensitive to vibrations in the cosmos and internally.

Pranayama is a method of refining the makeup of one's pranic body, one's physical body and also of one's mind. In this way, it is possible for a practitioner to become aware of new dimensions of existence. By making the mind calm and still, consciousness is allowed to shine through without distortion. In *Yoga Chudamani Upanishad* (v.89) it is written:

Chale vaate chalo binduh nishchale bhavet;
Yogee sthaanuttvamaapnoti tato vayum nirundhayet.

When the prana moves, the bindu also moves. When the prana remains steady, then the bindu is also steady. Thus the yogi becomes steadfast and firm. Therefore, the prana should be controlled.

Does the term 'pranayama' mean to expand, or to control the prana?

Swami Niranjanananda: Pranayama is a precise science which provides methods to understand the essence of prana and to guide it within oneself, as well as in the rest of creation. The medium of pranayama is the breath. The practices involve guiding the respiration beyond its normal limit: stretching it, speeding it up and slowing it down in order to experience the full range of respiration at both the gross and subtle levels.

The word 'pranayama' has two etymological explanations. Firstly, pranayama has been interpreted as a

17

combination of the words 'prana' and 'ayama'. The word *ayama* means 'expanding the dimension', so in the first sense pranayama means expanding the dimension of prana. Each person has abilities and limitations. Each person is involved in a routine, from morning until night. According to this routine and its activities, peaks and lows of energy are experienced. If one is able to increase the length of the peaks by expanding the quality of the prana shakti within, then there is less tiredness. The moment one energizes oneself with pranayama, there is an expansion of prana shakti. The area of pranic activity increases. This is one meaning of pranayama.

Another meaning of pranayama is controlling and guiding the flow of prana as it manifests through the senses and through the mind. The word *yama* means 'restraint' or 'control', so here 'prana' plus 'yama' refers to holding, restraining or controlling the prana shakti. One begins to hold on when it is realized that the energies are being wasted in useless pursuits of the senses which are not going to give satisfaction or happiness, instead withdrawing and focusing the attention on something else. That is holding back, withdrawing, restraining the association of the senses with the sense objects.

When one withdraws the prana shakti the senses become weak and then the corresponding part in the mind also loses its intensity. Obsessive desires become dissipated, not focussed. They lose their obsessive quality and simply become a desire which can be adjusted, accommodated and even manipulated. This aspect of restraining the prana shakti leads to the experience of pratyahara.

Prana is a force in constant motion: therefore, if prana-yama is understood as prana plus yama, the only way to control a moving force is by stopping it to the extent of complete cessation. Only then is one able to harness its power. This point of complete cessation is *kumbhaka*, or breath retention, whereby the force of prana is held, restrained and directed towards a specific purpose, the awakening of kundalini shakti and union with the divine. However, when pranayama is understood as prana plus ayama, it refers to a process of stretching, extending or expanding. In this context, pranayama is the process by which the internal pranic dimension is expanded, increased and held, thereby activating the prana in the body to a higher frequency.

What is the difference between the pranayama of hatha yoga and raja yoga?

Swami Sivananda: The practices of concentration and pranayama are interdependent. If pranayama is practised, there will be concentration. Similarly, natural pranayama follows the practice of concentration. A hatha yogi practices pranayama and then controls the mind. He rises from a lower to a higher level; whereas a raja yogi practices concentration and thus controls prana. He comes down from a higher level. They both meet on a common platform in the end. There are different practices for different temperaments: for some the practice of pranayama is easier to start with, for others the practice of concentration.

What is the raja yoga definition of pranayama?

Swami Satyananda: In raja yoga the definition of pranayama is explicit and clear: inhalation and exhalation is not pranayama. It says in Sage Patanjali's *Yoga Sutras* (2:49), that the gap between inhalation and exhalation is pranayama:

Tasminsati shvaasaprashvaasayor gativichchhedaha praanaayaamaha.

The asana having been done, pranayama is the cessation of the movement of inhalation and exhalation.

This means that kumbhaka or retention is pranayama. It must be remembered, however, that inhalation and exhalation are a part of retention, because in order to retain the breath, it has to be inhaled and it has to be exhaled.

What does Sage Patanjali mean when he says that retention of the breath is pranayama?

Swami Niranjanananda: In the *Yoga Sutras*, Sage Patanjali was not trying to say that just by closing the nostrils and retaining the breath one can attain enlightenment. However, controlling and moving the breath with a specific purpose, direction and aim is not pranayama. In the *Yoga Sutras* Sage Patanjali talks of three types of pranayama: i) breathing in, ii) breathing out, and iii) retaining the breath, holding the breath, not breathing. When he says pranayama is breathing in, one begins to think that he is talking of the physical process of breathing. But breath is not prana; breath is *shvasa*. Breathing is *shvasan kriya*, inhalation and exhalation.

When Sage Patanjali says that pranayama is breathing in, he is indicating a stage of perfection in which one is able to accumulate prana within oneself. When he says pranayama is breathing out, he is indicating a stage in which one is able to distribute that prana shakti for mental and spiritual growth. When he says pranayama is holding the breath, it indicates that there is no movement of prana, that prana has become stable.

Sage Patanjali has used the word pranayama to mean 'enlarging the dimension of prana'. Enlarging the dimension of prana is the literal meaning of pranayama. Retention, therefore, is the key as it allows a longer period for the assimilation of prana. Technically speaking therefore, pranayama is actually only retention.

Why has pranayama been considered secret, and even dangerous?

Swami Niranjanananda: Traditionally pranayama has been considered a very secret practice. In fact many aspects of yoga are considered to be secret due to lack of understanding. If something can be understood properly then it is not secret, but if it can't be understood then it is secret. This applies to pranayama. This is why there are books

20

on yoga by modern authors who say that pranayama is dangerous and should not be practised. One has to smile at such statements.

PRANA NIGRAHA

What is the process of pranayama?

Swami Niranjanananda: Pranayama begins as a system of regulating the breathing process, but ends with the awakening of the vital force within the body. The hatha yoga texts describe four aspects of pranayama: i) the process of inhalation, ii) the process of exhalation, iii) the process of internal retention, and iv), the process of external retention. Therefore, pranayama is related to the breath but the pranayamas that are generally done, such as nadi shodhana, bhastrika, bhramari, ujjayi, kapalbhati, sheetali, sheetkari or any other form, are not pranayamas in the real sense; they are *prana nigraha* techniques. The word *nigraha* means 'control'.

What is prana nigraha?

Swami Niranjanananda: The word *pranayama* is used freely nowadays; anybody who closes their nose says, "I am practising pranayama." But literally, classically and traditionally speaking that is not pranayama, it is shwas nigraha.

When one starts the practice of pranayama the first stage is control of the breath, which is called *shwas nigraha*. After that, when one has the ability to breathe in, breathe out and retain the breath in and out for 'x' number of seconds, it becomes prana nigraha, leading to pranayama. Traditionally, the ideal length of a breath is the length of *Gayatri* mantra which has twenty-four *matras*. These matras can be associated with twenty-four seconds. One breathes in for twenty-four seconds, holds the breath in for twenty-four seconds and then breathes out for twenty-four seconds. Perfecting the breath in this manner leads to entry into the dimension of prana.

21

What is the real practice of pranayama?

Swami Niranjanananda: In the practice of pranayama an important link is seen, that of impulses and stimulations. In the practice of bandhas another link is seen: energy, prana, moving in a different direction than normal. If one is able to understand the pranas, one's behaviour can be understood. The brain, the organs, the impulses and the pranic energy, intermingle with each other and go into a hyperactive, turbo mode. Just as in a computer one can change from twenty-five mega hertz to thirty-three by pressing the turbo button, in the same way, in the real practice of pranayama one can change the normal mode and go into turbo mode. Then what happens? Sparks begin to fly inside.

Pranayama in this context, however, does not refer to the breathing techniques with which people are familiar; those are the prana nigraha techniques. Yoga students have not yet practised pranayama. A fine distinction needs to be recognized between pranayama and the prana nigraha techniques that are being practised. When pranayama is practised, sparks begin to fly, and this hyper mode of the body is actually the tuning of the body, the harmonizing of the body with itself.

What is the distinction between prana nigraha and pranayama?

Swami Niranjanananda: After completing the practice of asana and coming to a mode of steadiness and harmony in the neuromuscular structure, there are five different stages of pranayama.

The first stage begins with learning how to breathe properly. The second stage is controlling and directing the breath. The third stage is understanding the states of body and mind in relation to the breath. The fourth stage is becoming aware of the impulses which are being generated in the neurocellular structure of the body, becoming aware of the physical and the pranic link between the body and the brain. The fifth stage is allowing the pranas to dominate the functions of the body.

The first three stages of pranayama are known as prana nigraha and the last two are the actual pranayama. In the fourth and fifth stages of pranayama, the perineal space, the thoracic space and the head space are linked in one unit. Fusion of pranas takes place, and the plural is used here, because prana is not one.

Why is pranayama based on breath control?

Swami Niranjanananda: The hatha yoga tradition places a lot of emphasis on the practices of pranayama. Although the practices of pranayama are few in number, much explanation has been given to the purpose, function and benefits of the pranayamas. In *Gheranda Samhita* (5:45–46) just eight pranayamas are listed:

> *Evamvidhaam naadee shuddhim kritvaa naadeem vishodhayet;*
> *Dridhobhootvaasanam kritvaa praanaayaamam samaacharet.*

> *Sahitah sooryabhedashcha ujjaayee sheetalee tathaa;*
> *Bhastrikaa bhraamaree moorchchhaa kevalee chaashtakumbhakaah.*

> After purifying the nadis, sit in a steady asana (posture) and prepare for pranayama. (45)

> There are eight types of pranayama: sahita, surya bheda, ujjayi, sheetali, bhastrika, bhramari, moorchha and kevali. (46)

Normally pranayama is associated with breath control, however, it is not actually breath control. *Prana* means 'prana' and *ayama* means 'dimension' or *kshetr*, therefore *pranayama* means 'awareness of the pranic dimension'. But how do we become aware of this pranic dimension? By following the breath, which is the external form of prana, the life force.

If there is no control over the breath, then there cannot be any control over the movement of prana shakti. In normal life, if one stops breathing, the pranas also stop, their movement dies. There comes a time, however, when through the combined practice of *pooraka*, inhalation; *rechaka*, exhalation and *kumbhaka*, retention, it is possible to awaken the subtle prana shakti. At that time the breath is disassociated from prana shakti.

PURPOSE OF PRANAYAMA

Why is pranayama important in spiritual life?

Swami Sivananda: Prana and mind are intimately related to each other. If prana is controlled, the mind will be controlled. If the mind is controlled, the prana will be automatically controlled. Prana is related to mind, and through it to will, and through will to the individual soul, and through the individual soul to the Supreme Soul.

How does pranayama purify the body and mind?

Swami Sivananda: Just as a goldsmith removes the impurities of gold by heating it in the blazing furnace and vigorously blowing the blowpipe, so also the student of yoga should remove the various impurities of his body and mind by blowing his lungs through the practice of pranayama. Just as it takes a long time, patience and perseverance to tame a lion, an elephant or tiger, so also this prana has to be gradually tamed. Then it will come under perfect control.

What are the main purposes of pranayama?

Swami Satyananda: The first purpose of pranayama is to supply energy to the nervous system. The second purpose is to awaken kundalini. The third purpose of pranayama is to awaken the sleeping centres of the brain. It is said that thought influences prana, and prana influences thought.

According to the yogic texts the purpose of pranayama is to handle the mind. The scriptures on yoga make it clear – mind and prana are interacting. When the mind is restless it affects the prana; when the mind is peaceful, calm and tranquil, there is automatic equipoise in the prana. The reverse is also true. When the pranas are agitated the mind is agitated. When the pranas are controlled, the mind is controlled. In Sage Patanjali's *Yoga Sutras* (2:53) it is said:

Dharanasu cha yogyata manasah.

And fitness of the mind for concentration (develops through pranayama).

Therefore, if pranayama is correctly followed, one can attain the highest steps in yoga.

What was the original purpose and experience of pranayama?

Swami Niranjanananda: The science of pranayama was developed by highly evolved yogis through an intuitive and experiential understanding of prana and its influence on the human mechanism at various levels. The breath was used to access the pranic field, to attain balance in the body and control of the mind. The practices would render the body-mind instrument capable of experiencing higher states of consciousness, so that the ultimate union with the transcendental reality could be experienced. In *Hatharatnavali* (3:79) it is written:

Chale vaate chalam sarvam nishchale nishchite hathabandhanam.

When vata (air) is not steady, everything is not steady. When vata becomes steady, then only mastery of hatha is acquired.

What are the fruits of pranayama?

Swami Sivananda: Pranayama is an exact science. It is the fourth limb of raja yoga. The fundamental aim of pranayama is to unite the prana and the apana and to take the united prana-apana slowly towards the crown of the head. The fruit of pranayama is the awakening of the sleeping kundalini shakti.

Through the practice of pranayama the prana leaves the passages of ida and pingala nadis, forces itself through the mouth of sushumna, and enters therein. Sushumna is the only passage through which, when the prana passes, the light of *jnana*, wisdom, is kindled. When the prana moves through sushumna, the mind enters a thoughtless region. All the seeds of karma in the yogi are thereby burnt away.

All the pranas are united during kumbhaka or retention of breath. The yogi offers the oblation of the senses into the fire of prana. Therefore the practice of pranayama is indispensable to the yogi. In the *Yoga Chudamani Upanishad* (v.92) it is written:

Alpakaalabhayaadbrahmaa praanaayaamaparo bhavet;
Yogino munayashchaiva tatah praanaannirodhayet.

Even Brahma, fearing a short life span, became a practitioner of pranayama. Therefore, yogis and munis should also control the prana.

Just as it takes a long time, patience and perseverance to tame a lion, an elephant or tiger, so also the prana must be tamed gradually. Then it will come under perfect control. Only advanced students will attain these fruits of pranayama.

What are the effects of controlling prana through the practice of pranayama?

Swami Sivananda: The process by which prana is controlled by regulation of breath is pranayama. Psychic cure, telepathy, thought-reading and other siddhis are the effects of the control of prana. It is through pranayama that one can control one's circumstances and character, and consciously harmonize the individual life with the cosmic life.

Is physical and mental wellbeing the purpose of practising pranayama?

Swami Niranjanananda: In general, pranayama practice helps to resolve physical and mental disturbances. As the

26

art of correct breathing is mastered, respiratory problems come to an end. As one becomes capable of controlling the breath, initially by simply observing it, many mental problems like anger, despondency and worry cease. The practitioner of pranayama will certainly experience many benefits at the physical level. These effects have been documented scientifically, and it has been observed that pranayama influences almost all the organs and physiological systems.

When these effects are experienced in daily life it is sometimes thought that managing physical and mental health is the only aim of pranayama, but when the rishis discovered the science of pranayama they did not have yoga therapy in mind. Although the practices have innumerable physical benefits, the therapeutic aspect of pranayama is an incidental by-product. The main objective of pranayama, however, is to balance the interacting processes of the pranic and mental forces for awakening the higher centres of human consciousness: the real purpose of pranayama is to awaken the pranas, chakras and kundalini.

What is the relevance of pranayama to tantra?
Swami Satyananda: Prana denotes constancy, it is a force in constant motion. Prana is the vital life force and pranayama is the process by which the internal pranic store is increased. It is a technique through which the quantity of prana in the body is activated to a higher frequency.

In yogic terminology it is said that whatever is manifest is the *sthoola roopa*, or gross form of the subtle, cosmic energy, known as prana. In yoga and tantra there is an eternal truth: the basis of existence depends on two forces, *Shiva* and *Shakti*, or consciousness and energy. Ultimately they are not two forces but one – Shakti, or prana, is the creative force of consciousness, or Shiva. The purpose of hatha yoga is to realize Shiva, consciousness, by means of Shakti, prana

SCIENCE AND PRANAYAMA

Are the benefits of pranayama recognized by science?

Swami Niranjanananda: Medical science has done a significant amount of research on the effects of pranayama over the last few decades. Once translated as 'breathing exercises', pranayama is now recognized by scientists throughout the world as a means of invigorating, enhancing and accelerating the revitalizing processes of the body.

Studies have been published on pranayama research undertaken in countries such as Australia, Russia, Turkey, Germany, USA, India and others. These studies give modern understanding of an ancient science which arose through intuition and depth of experience.

What have scientific studies revealed about the effects of conscious breathing on the brain?

Swami Satyananda: The brain consists of the frontal brain and the posterior brain. The posterior brain is the instinctive, or primitive brain. The frontal brain is the seat of total consciousness. When one breathes without awareness, the breath is registered in the posterior brain. This is called involuntary breathing. When one is aware of breathing and consciously witnessing the whole process, it is called voluntary breathing and it is registered by the conscious brain, the frontal brain.

This difference seems to be simple, but its effect is great. Throughout life, most people breathe unconsciously, just like animals and children. A few people who have started practising yoga are the exception. The moment one becomes aware of the breathing and begins to conduct and control the breath in a particular fashion, the frontal brain immediately registers the influence. This fact has been revealed by scientific experiments and has led to the conclusion that conscious breathing has an entirely different effect on the brain than unconscious breathing. Through unconscious breathing the whole body is supplied with prana, but this supply is insufficient for its evolution and growth.

This means that pranayama is not only a breathing exercise or breath control, it is a system for training the different centres in the brain. An example of voluntary breathing is alternate nostril breathing. Scientific studies have observed that when one breathes in the left nostril, activity increases in the right hemisphere of the brain, and when one breathes in the right nostril, activity increases in the left hemisphere of the brain. When the breath is held, both hemispheres of the brain are equalized.

It has also been observed that the breath which goes through the left nostril has a slightly lower temperature than the breath which goes through the right. This concurs with the yogic understanding that the left nostril is related to *ida nadi*, the flow of mental energy, while the right nostril is related to *pingala nadi*, the flow of vital energy. Ida is the lunar force, which is cool, while pingala is the solar force, which is hot.

In scientific experiments related to stress, ECG (electro cardiograph) and EEG (electro encephalograph) are used to record heart rhythm and brainwaves, and GSR (galvanic skin response) to measure electrical activity of the skin. It has been found that the practice of pranayama results in a synchronous flow of alpha, delta or theta waves, which harmonizes the activity of the brain. The tensions recorded during periods of beta activity reduce when alpha, theta or delta waves replace the beta activity. When the alpha waves manifest in the brain tensions in the body are lowered and the heart becomes free from stress-related pressure.

How does the practice of pranayama affect the brainwaves?
Swami Niranjanananda: Biofeedback systems have shown that the frequency of the brainwaves can be wilfully changed by learning how to relax the muscles, control the breath, or divert the mind from the most immediate problem to another experience. This is exactly what happens when

pranayama is practised during a state of mental conflict, tension and frustration. There is a gradual reduction of beta waves, but that does not mean that alpha waves automatically increase. There are practices of pranayama in which one bypasses the alpha, theta and delta waves. From beta one goes straight to shoonya – no activity!

Many researchers and swamis have conducted such experiments. I was fortunate enough to see the experiment which showed that a pranayama practitioner could go straight from beta waves into the state of shoonya without passing through the alpha, delta and theta phases. The subject of the experiment was the same sannyasin, Swami Nadabrahmananda, who stopped breathing for forty five minutes while placed in a cage. Needless to say, this is a great achievement.

What have scientific investigations revealed about the effect of pranayama on the physical body, the brain and mental health?

Swami Niranjanananda: The practice of pranayama has a direct effect on the functioning of the intricate, sophisticated functions of the brain. When the yogis investigated the possibility of an independent method to develop the silent areas of the mind and brain in order to transcend the limiting barriers of the human personality, they discovered pranayama. It is possible to understand this process through modern scientific principles as well.

Scientific investigations into pranayama have revealed that practitioners have decreased adrenocortical response to ongoing stress, which equates to an increased ability to resist stress. The brain's activity is dominated by alpha waves during pranayama and there is lowered oxygen consumption and use of the full lung capacity. Practitioners also showed less neuroticism, decreased mental fatigue, improved awareness in daily life, cardiac and respiratory function improved and there was a marked increase in immunity. Conscious breathing has a calming effect on the mind. Even simple breath awareness is an effective method of quietening a tense mind. The more complex breathing techniques of pranayama influence the brain even more deeply.

The bandhas used during pranayama stretch and squeeze specific areas of the body, restoring optimal nervous connections to the vital organs, including the endocrine glands. The endocrine glands related to these nerves are activated, resulting in better functioning. The endocrine glands influence the behaviour, reactions, interpretations, and the so-called natural responses. Since these glands are often overactive, pranayama allows them to work properly and harmoniously for better health and physical wellbeing.

Certain pranayamas alternately stimulate and inhibit the parasympathetic and sympathetic nervous systems. There are billions of cells in the brain which exist in a chaotic order, shown as random brainwave activity when measured on an EEG machine. These cells are oscillating forms of energy or shakti. The chaos in the mind is also a result of the millions of archetypes that exist as unorganized geometric patterns influencing one's actions, thoughts, decisions, feelings and awareness as a whole.

Conscious breathing has been shown to engage the cerebral cortex and stimulate the more evolved areas of the brain. The regular practice of pranayama over a period of time reinforces the cortical control of the breath, with profound effects on one's wellbeing. During conscious control of the breath, the cerebral cortex bypasses the respiratory centre in the primitive brain stem. Impulses from the cortex also affect adjoining areas of the brain concerned with emotions. The involvement of the cerebral cortex in conscious breathing causes the cortex to develop and allows the individual to enter higher stages of the evolutionary cycle.

Pranayama practice also influences the higher functions of the brain, such as cognition, perception and memory. The cumulative effect of pranayama is that the mind becomes steady like a candle flame in a still room.

What research been conducted into the effects of prana-yama on cardiac health?

Swami Niranjanananda: In 1968, the Bihar School of Yoga was asked by the Health Ministry of the Government of India to conduct research on coronary diseases and yoga. About one thousand patients suffering from cardiac disorders such as angina, myocardial infarction and other cardiac diseases were referred to yoga and pranayama practices. At the end of the study period, it was found that the practice of pranayama had helped each and every patient, but especially those suffering from angina and ischemia. Many other research studies have verified that pranayama is extremely beneficial for the heart. The practices minimize the stress put on the cardiac system by day-to-day life. Breathing with slow, deep and long breaths gives rest to the heart. Many heart conditions can be managed through pranayama.

Pranayama gives proper training to the coronary behaviour and this has another implication for the spiritual aspirant. When the practitioner enters the state of meditation having practised pranayama, there is no stress on the heart, and the body is able to withstand the higher states of consciousness without any adverse effect.

What evidence is there about the benefits of pranayama on general health and wellbeing?

Swami Niranjanananda: The yogis who expounded on the practices of pranayama knew that a sustained and systematic practice would relieve the practitioner of various diseases. In *Hatha Yoga Pradipika* (2:17) it says:

Hikkaa shvaasashcha kaasashcha shirahkarnaakshivedanaah;
Bhavanti vividhaa rogaah pavanasya prakopatah.

Hiccups, asthma, coughs, headache, ear and eye pain, and various other diseases are due to disturbances of the vital air.

In the former Soviet Union, scientists conducted research into the effects of pranayama on resistance and immunity. Astronauts were sent into space after being trained in pranayama and it was found that they were able to endure the altered external environment much more easily than those who had not received the training. It was concluded that the practice of pranayama improves the resistance of all the systems that defend the body from extraneous factors.

Numerous other studies on pranayama have established that the practices reduce stress and hypertension, normalize blood pressure (both high and low), alleviate heart disease, increase vitality and lung capacity, and balance the relationship between the brain hemispheres. It has also been found that pranayama results in a synchronous flow of alpha, delta and theta waves, which harmonizes the brain and heart activity.

What research has been done on specific pranayama techniques?

Swami Niranjanananda: Research on specific pranayama techniques has consistently shown that many benefits flow from their practice.

Nadi shodhana pranayama is one of the most important practices in yoga. In 2002, the Yoga Research Foundation (YRF), Munger, India, undertook a research project to study some of the basic psycho-physiological effects of nadi shodhana pranayama on healthy subjects. 22 resident students of Bihar School of Yoga aged from 19 to 62 years were studied for a period of six months. The parameters of the research were: performance speed in repetitive mathematical tasks, breath holding time (BHT), peak expiratory flow, systolic and diastolic blood pressure, pulse rate, effects on swara and pranic experiences.

Performance speed in the mathematical tasks increased and BHT and peak expiratory flow showed improvement in the whole group. In terms of swara, significant change was recorded in the balanced flow in the two nostrils. Pranic experiences at ajna were more noticeable as compared to those at mooladhara.

In another study conducted by YRF in 2007 on 30 hypertensive adults in Bhopal it was found that the practice of nadi shodhana pranayama for one month (ratio of 1:1) brought down both systolic and diastolic blood pressures.

YRF also conducted a study in 2006 in Bhopal on the effects of ujjayi pranayama. 22 asthmatics, 11 hypertensives and 7 healthy adults practised ujjayi for over one month for five minutes every day. The asthmatics gained the most from the practice. The amount of oxygen assimilated into the blood increased from 0.75% up to a 5% (maximum), the average being 2% – a significant percentage clinically.

Research on bhramari was carried out on 112 pregnant women in 1993 by Munger Hospital, India, in cooperation with Bihar School of Yoga. Results compared with a control group showed normal blood pressure in all, lower number of miscarriages, fewer premature births, 25% shorter labour, reduced pain during labour, reduced incidence of Caesarean section, greater average weight for newborns and no newborns suffered lack of oxygen at birth. Bhramari has also been shown to provide multiple benefits in surgical patients and there is ample evidence that bhramari works as a stress reducer.

Bhastrika and kapalbhati, known as vitalizing pranayamas, have been shown to provide significant exercise for the respiratory muscles with only a mild to moderate overall body work output. It has also been recorded that while practising kapalbhati, bhastrika, surya bheda and moorchha pranayamas, there are extra impulses in the central autonomous system, resulting in increased activity in the brain. In yogic terms, this indicates the awakening of sushumna. This is supported by the YRF (2004) study, which showed a change of swara to sushumna in most cases after the practice.

CATEGORIES OF PRANAYAMA

What is meant by the different categories of pranayama?

Swami Satyananda: More recently, pranayama has been categorized into balancing practices, vitalizing practices and tranquillizing practices. Of course the overall effects of any pranayama are tranquillizing, however, some particularly activate pranic movement and the sympathetic nervous system, while others pacify or cool the system. The vitalizing practices rapidly create heat in the physical and subtle bodies, and such practices are more suitable for middle to advanced sadhakas. Beginners should always start with nadi shodhana to balance the breath and the flow of ida and pingala nadis, which relate to the parasympathetic and sympathetic nervous systems.

Tranquillizing pranayama practices are those which pacify the body and mind. They simultaneously increase the pranic flow and arouse awareness of the subtle vibration of energy. Such forms of pranayama stimulate activity in the parasympathetic and central nervous systems. These techniques should be performed once the pranic flow is balanced. Therefore, they generally involve breathing through both the nostrils.

How does one know which pranayama to practise?

Swami Satyananda: The pranayamas are of various types, some for people who have a restless mind and others for people who have a calm and quiet mind. Some people are naturally introverted and some are extroverted. Therefore, the pranayama to be practised should be selected according to the type of person.

There is a pranayama known as bhastrika, in which the breathing is made rapid. This pranayama is for people who have an active, restless mind. People who are restless cannot keep their mind at one point, even for one second. If they try to concentrate on one point, they find after a few seconds that their mind is thinking of something else and they didn't know it. Bhastrika pranayama is important and effective for these people.

For others, nadi shodhana pranayama, alternate nostril breathing, is important, and five rounds should be practised before meditation. A ratio between inhalation and exhalation must be established, as only then will it affect the brain. How to breathe and what ratio to maintain should be learnt personally from one's teacher.

Are different pranayamas suitable for different people?
Swami Satyananda: There are many variations of pranayama although there are only three main processes of breathing. These are inspiration, retention and exhalation. In the various pranayamas any of these breathing processes may be overemphasized or underemphasized.

These variations are intended for different types of people. Those suffering from hypertension should not do quick breathing, whereas those who are suffering from nervous depressions resulting in lethargy, laziness and low blood pressure, must practise quick inspiration and expiration. Those who wish to improve the balance between the parasympathetic and sympathetic nervous systems should breathe in and out very, very slowly. And those who wish to have control of the autonomic nervous system should learn retention of the breath.

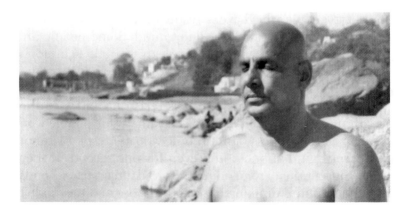

2

Breath

IMPORTANCE OF THE BREATH

How is the breath linked to the experience of life?
Swami Satyananda: The breath is the most vital process of the body. It influences the activities of each and every cell and, most importantly, is intimately linked with the performance of the brain. Human beings breathe about 15 times per minute and 21,600 times per day. Respiration fuels the burning of oxygen and glucose, producing energy to power every muscular contraction, glandular secretion and mental process. The breath is intimately linked to all aspects of human experience.

How does control of the breath influence the various dimensions of life?
Swami Sivananda: By controlling the act of breathing one can efficiently control all the various motions in the body and the different nerve currents that run through the body. One can easily and quickly control and develop body, mind and soul through breath control or the control of prana. It is through pranayama that one's circumstances and character can be controlled and the individual life can consciously be harmonized with the cosmic life.

The breath, directed by thought under the control of the will, is a vitalizing, regenerating force which can be used consciously for self development, for healing many incurable diseases both in oneself and in others and, for other various useful purposes.

The breath is within easy reach at every moment of life. Use it judiciously. Many yogins of yore, like Sri Jnanadeva, Trailinga Swami, Ramalinga Swami and others, used the breath and through it, this force, the prana, in a variety of ways.

Realize the occult inner life powers which underlie the breath. Practise pranayama as prescribed. Become a yogi and radiate joy, light and power all around. *Pranavadins*, or hatha yogis, consider prana tattwa to be superior to *manas tattwa*, the mind principle. They say prana is present even when the mind is absent during sleep. Hence prana plays a more vital part than the mind.

Why is it important to know one's breath?
Swami Niranjanananda: Nothing is closer than one's own breath. It is tangible, believable, understandable and controllable. The gentle inhalation and exhalation is sustaining and calming, it affects one's thoughts and is itself affected by one's activities, emotions and thoughts. Everyone experiences this daily, yet the breath is often ignored or forgotten.

In the practices of pranayama, a deep familiarity with the breath develops. Knowledge of the respiratory system aids and enhances the practices, helping bring a better understanding of their physiological parameters.

Why does hatha yoga give so much attention to the breath?
Swami Niranjanananda: The breath has a close relationship with the body. Whether doing asana, pranayama, dhauti or any hatha yoga practice, it is essential to have control over the breath, as according to yoga the breath is a mirror of the mental and emotional state. If the mind and emotions are restless or scattered, it can be observed in the breath. If a person is lying down and has many thoughts going through the mind and cannot stop those thoughts, the breathing will be rapid, short and unsteady. The breathing process will be

mainly in the upper portion of the lungs and unconsciously the person will be longing for a deep calming breath. Alternatively, if the breathing pattern of a person who is calm, not distressed or restless, is observed, the breath will be found to be calm.

According to yoga there is also a relationship between the breath and the pranic body. Many people believe that if the breath is retained for a longer period, they might even die, but this is an incorrect concept. If the breath is withheld forcibly without practice, the face will turn black, brown, blue, and finally one must breathe, or indeed, death would result. It is quite possible, however, for a siddha yogi to function without the breath for up to half an hour and still be alive. The general public sees this as a *siddhi*, an accomplishment, but in the tradition, restraining the breath is not thought of as a siddhi, but as a capacity of the body. It is also possible to hold air inside the body for up to forty minutes, one hour or longer. There are many things the body can do, but it is essential to understand the body and recognize its capacity.

Prana can exist without breath. The breath has a relationship with *prana shakti*, the life force or energy, but prana is different from the breath. The difference is that prana shakti is present in the physical body in the form of heat, energy and brilliance. The inner heat, or body temperature, is an activity of prana shakti. If one does not breathe in for two minutes, it makes no difference, but if prana does not exist inside the body even for a second, one instantly dies. In its subtle state, prana shakti exists in the form of activity. That is why there is an experience of restlessness, excitement or activity in emotion, in the expression of love, attachment, attraction, anger, desire, lust and craving.

In one sense, prana shakti is even behind the thoughts, but its form is changed and it is called *chitta shakti*. Prana shakti is physical and extroverted, whereas chitta shakti is internal, mental, emotional and intellectual. Hatha yoga makes an effort to awaken and balance the forces of

39

chitta shakti and prana shakti in the body; that is why the breathing process has been emphasized in hatha yoga. External practices are performed with the body, but in order to vibrate and awaken the inner shakti it is important to have control over the breath; this is an internal process.

How does one develop awareness of prana?

Swami Niranjanananda: Yoga says to start with breath awareness. The moods and states of the mind are reflected in the way one breathes in and out. If one is agitated, nervous, tense and angry, the breathing pattern will be shallow. The breath will be short and will remain in the upper thoracic region. When one is relaxed, the breath is deep, long and relaxed. Sometimes in deep states of relaxation the breath cannot even be noticed, it is so gentle. Therefore, yogis use the breath to regulate and harmonize the physical systems, like the nervous system. They use the breath to tranquillize the functions of the mind. In this way, through the breath, awareness of prana is developed.

BREATH AWARENESS AND MIND

What is the purpose of breath awareness?

Swami Satyananda: Concentration on breath is one of the most powerful methods of introverting the restless mind yet most people do not even know that they breathe. From birth until death everyone breathes; unbroken breathing is life. One can breathe voluntarily and involuntarily, consciously and unconsciously, but mostly it is unconscious. The whole night one breathes but doesn't know it. The whole day one breathes, but doesn't know it. Is it not surprising that the breathing process, which is so intimate, so important, so close, is something people don't know about? Become aware of the breath, because this is the way.

Observing one's breath for ten or fifteen minutes every morning gives absolute tranquillity of mind. The breath is gross and tangible. It can be felt and understood. It can be

40

concentrated on, and each inspiration and expiration can be observed. It may not be possible to do this for one hour, but at least it can be done for ten minutes, because the breath is not something abstract. Breath is connected with the life force and when one breathes in and breathes out, this should be observed. Yoga starts with pranic awareness, and pranic awareness starts with breath awareness.

Why is awareness of the natural breath practised?
Swami Satyananda: Awareness of the natural breath is a simple technique which introduces practitioners to their own respiratory system and breathing patterns. It is very relaxing and may be practised at any time. Awareness of the breathing process is itself sufficient to slow down the respiratory rate and establish a more relaxed rhythm.

Why is awareness of the natural breath important?
Swami Niranjanananda: The breath should become a part of one's constant awareness. The first step towards achieving this is to simply become aware of the breathing process. Without awareness, nothing can be achieved in regard to the breath. Although the breathing process continues twenty-four hours a day, one is neither aware nor in control of this vital process. Simple techniques can be used to develop increased awareness of the breathing process.

What happens when consciousness is directed to the breath?
Swami Niranjanananda: Breathing is a deep internal process that can be used to focus attention. The problem in meditation is that a focus is needed for one's attention: the breath is a place on which to put the attention.

If consciousness is directed to any part of the body, it will enliven the prana in that part. As soon as the mind is connected with an outer or inner part of the body, the outer cortex is linked with the inner brain. Deep, internal connections start to be created.

41

What is the effect of conscious breathing on the brain?

Swami Niranjanananda: The breath is perhaps the only physiological process that can be either voluntary or involuntary. One can breathe consciously and control the breathing process or one can breathe reflexively or unconsciously.

If the breath is unconscious, it falls under the control of primitive parts of the brain, where emotions, thoughts and feelings of which one has little or no awareness become involved. However, the moment one starts to breathe consciously, the frontal brain registers the breath, allowing control of the different hemispheres of the brain.

How does conscious breathing influence the mind?

Swami Satyananda: Although breathing is mainly an unconscious process, conscious control of it may be taken at any time. Consequently, it forms a bridge between the conscious and unconscious areas of the mind. Through the practice of pranayama, the energy trapped in neurotic, unconscious mental patterns may be released for use in more creative and joyful activity.

What is the relationship between breath, prana and the mind?

Swami Sivananda: Prana is the sum total of all energy that is manifest in the universe. It is the vital force. Heat, light, electricity, magnetism are all manifestations of prana. Breath is the external manifestation of prana. By exercising control over this gross breath, the subtle pranas inside can be controlled.

Just as there is a nervous system in the gross physical body, there is a nervous system in the astral body. The nervous system of the physical body is the *sthoola*, gross, prana. The nervous system of the astral body is the *sukshma*, subtle, prana. There is an intimate connection and interaction between these two pranas. It is the sukshma prana that is connected with the mind.

42

Control of the subtle, psychic prana can be attained by restraining the breath. That is the reason why pranayama is prescribed for controlling prana. Prana is the overcoat of the mind. If the prana can be controlled, the mind can be controlled. Prana is related to mind; through mind to the will; through will to the individual soul, and through this to the Supreme Being.

Does the breathing pattern reflect the state of mind?

Swami Niranjanananda: Incorrect and irregular breathing often reflects various disturbances in the body and mind. Everyone is familiar with the disruption in the breathing pattern associated with pain or powerful emotions. A sob of grief, a startled gasp, and the deep trembling breaths of anger are well known examples of how emotion affects the breathing.

This process also works the other way around. Correct breathing profoundly improves one's physical and mental wellbeing. Therefore, conscious breathing is a prerequisite of pranayama. This makes it possible to correct disturbed breathing habits. Quick, shallow breathing is detrimental to physical and emotional wellbeing, integration and balance. One should become conscious of the breath and learn to maintain the normal breathing rate of fifteen breaths per minute. If one relaxes the body, stops worrying, and becomes aware of the breath for a minute or so, the breathing rate will drop down to fifteen. In order to develop conscious breathing, one must free the mind from emotional tension.

Respiration begins with the nose, and the breath in the nostrils is closely related to many subtle balances in the body-mind system; therefore, attention should be paid to ensuring its efficient operation. In pranayama, all breathing should be through the nose except where otherwise specified.

Does science recognize the link between breath and the mind?

Swami Niranjanananda: It seems that a link is slowly being recognized between the breath, the brain and mental states.

43

Scientists talk about breath rates indicating states of mind and emotion.

If one is internally peaceful the breath is long, slow and deep. Additionally, swara yoga states that if a person is relaxed, the length of the breath is so many *angulas*, finger widths. For a person who is tense or agitated, the length of the breath is a different number of finger widths; it becomes short, shallow and rapid. This principle has already been explained by swara yoga, and yet people today are only beginning to rediscover and apply it.

Just as today scientists are able to see a link between the breath, the brain and mental states, in the future, if this topic is studied more deeply, a link will be shown between the breath, the brain, the mind, prana and consciousness.

Why is pranayama said to be the most important technique of yoga?

Swami Niranjanananda: Much research has been done into the effect of breath and mantra on the human brain and mind. The breath is considered to be the mirror of one's mental state. When one is at rest, when one is peaceful, the breath is slower and more gentle. When one is under stress, the breath comes in short, shallow gasps, the length is reduced, and there is lack of control over the autonomic nervous system. If one simply observes the breath and combines a mantra with it, positive changes are quickly experienced; it is realized that breath and mantra are powerful tools to manage mental, emotional and psychic stress.

Although pranayama is a simple technique of inhalation and exhalation, internal breath retention and external breath retention, many physiological and psychological changes take place within the body, and the practitioner needs to become aware of them. Through the breath, the function of the nervous and cardiovascular systems and the brain can be altered, inducing a state of relaxation. Or conversely, via the breath a state of tension can be induced in the body and brain.

The process of inhalation creates some physical resistance, and this resistance or tension is not limited to the body but also affects the mind. Exhalation eliminates that tension, that build up of energy, and a state of tranquillity is reached by observing the breath. By means of the breath, the level of tension can be controlled, whether it is muscular, nervous or emotional.

The practices of pranayama are the most effective ones for managing imbalances in the nervous system, the brain and the mind. Pranayama links the nervous system with the brain, and the brain with the mind, the physical with the subtle. It links these three areas of existence together. Therefore, pranayama is the most important aspect of yoga.

CORRECT BREATHING

What is meant by correct breathing?
Swami Satyananda: Most people breathe incorrectly, using only a small part of their lung capacity. The breathing is then generally shallow, depriving the body of oxygen and prana essential to its good health. The first practices taught to pranayama students are preparatory techniques which introduce correct breathing habits. In addition, they help focus the awareness on the breathing process, which is otherwise normally ignored.

Although it takes some time to learn, it is possible to control the actions of respiration. Once the breathing has been corrected, one feels much better. When one breathes in, the stomach should inflate; when one breathes out the stomach should contract. Abdominal contraction and abdominal inflation should be synchronized with the breathing process. This is seen in all animals. Observe a dog or cat or any other animal.

The breath is both gross and subtle. The gross breath is perceptible and the subtle breath is imperceptible. When the breath becomes subtle it improves the quality of awareness.

The ingoing and outgoing breath should be uniform. It should not be thick or thin, broken or in waves.

How does incorrect breathing affect one's health?

Swami Satyananda: A person's health depends on the way they breathe and most people do not know how to breathe. If breathing is incorrect, there will be a tendency towards disease. Many people breathe only from the chest. Others contract their stomach during inhalation and expand it during exhalation. This is totally wrong. Before learning pranayama, the breathing must be corrected.

Why does yoga teach correct breathing?

Swami Satyananda: Before learning pranayama, yoga students must develop sensitivity to the respiratory process and retrain the muscles of the pulmonary cavity, enhancing their vital capacity and preparing them for pranayama.

Rhythmic, deep and slow respiration stimulates and is stimulated by calm, content, states of mind. Irregular breathing disrupts the rhythms of the brain and leads to physical, emotional and mental blocks. These, in turn, lead to inner conflict, an unbalanced personality, a disordered lifestyle, and disease. Pranayama establishes regular breathing patterns, breaking this negative cycle and reversing the debilitating process. It does so by giving one control of the breath and re-establishing the natural, relaxed rhythms of the body and mind.

What are the physical advantages of breathing deeply and slowly?

Swami Satyananda: Deep breathing allows maximum intake for each respiration and slow breathing allows optimum exchange of oxygen and carbon dioxide. Time is required to transfer oxygen from the lungs to the blood, and for carbon dioxide in the blood to be transferred into the lungs for expulsion into the air. If one breathes rapidly, then the optimum oxygen and carbon dioxide exchange is not reached in the lungs. If the respiration is slow then the optimum transfer can be achieved. This is why depth and speed of breathing are so important in relation to each other.

Why is the science of breathing so important for day to day wellbeing?

Swami Satyananda: Pranayama has a two-sided effect. It helps to keep the physical apparatus pure and in good order, and also to control, regulate and channel the mental-emotional being of man. Pranayama involves controlled, rhythmic and regular breathing. Prana is the gross manifestation in the physical body of the subtle, universal, cosmic force. It is this cosmic energy that gives life to all sentient beings. Pranayama is the technique of conservation and distribution of this life force.

While inhaling, oxygen is taken in, and while exhaling carbon dioxide is discharged. Oxygenation of the system makes the body pure, light and active. Unless the science of breathing is properly understood and correctly practised, there is a likelihood of imbalance in breathing, which may result in various types of mental and emotional conflicts and impulsiveness.

The world with its innumerable joys and sorrows makes a violent impact upon the individual and one often fails to find a realistic way of adjusting to life. The effect of prana on the human being and the correlation between the mind and the body are fully realized in yoga.

How does correct breathing influence the length of life?

Swami Satyananda: In addition to influencing the quality of life, the length or quantity of life is also dictated by the rhythm of respiration. The ancient yogis and rishis studied nature in great detail. They noticed that animals with a slow breath rate such as pythons, elephants and tortoises have long lifespans, whereas those with a fast breathing rate such as birds, dogs and rabbits live for only a few years. From this observation they realized the importance of slow breathing for increasing the human lifespan.

Those who breathe in short, quick gasps are likely to have a shorter lifespan than those who breathe slowly and deeply. On the physical level, this is because respiration is directly related to the heart. A slow breathing rate keeps the heart stronger and better nourished and contributes to a longer life. Deep breathing also increases the absorption of energy by pranamaya kosha, enhancing dynamism, vitality and general wellbeing.

What is paradoxical breathing?

Swami Niranjanananda: The gasping breath or the para-doxical breath is another method of breathing outside the domain of the three natural methods of breathing. It manifests when the need to stimulate the sympathetic nervous system is most intense. One inhales so deeply and quickly that the abdominal wall moves in during inhalation rather than out. This is what occurs in a state of shock. For example, if one takes an ice-cold shower on a winter morning the mouth will probably open and suck air in with a gasp at the first contact with the water.

This is called paradoxical breathing because the ab-dominal wall moves in rather than out during inhalation, and out rather than in during exhalation. Paradoxical breathing stimulates the sympathetic nervous system even more than thoracic breathing. If one were to breathe in this way for even 10–15 breaths, one would immediately feel nervous and jumpy, for it gives an immediate jolt of adrenalin causing the fight or flight reaction. It is usually seen only in a state of acute anxiety.

How can the breath be corrected?

Swami Niranjanananda: The first step in relearning proper breathing is to master abdominal breathing. Some may find it difficult at first, but with practice it becomes automatic and natural. Abdominal breathing should be practised first in shavasana, then in a sitting or standing position.

BASIC BREATHING METHODS

What is rhythmic breathing?

Swami Sivananda: Breathing in men and women is generally irregular. The practice of rhythmic breathing brings the feeling of having enjoyed a good rest. When the units of exhalation and inhalation are the same, or are in some other regular ratio, that is rhythmic breathing. It harmonizes the whole system. Rhythmic breathing harmonizes the physical body, mind and senses, and soothes tired nerves. Full repose and calmness is experienced with this type of breathing. The bubbling emotions subside and the surging impulses calm down.

The duration of inhalation and exhalation can gradually be increased but the duration should never be increased until there is definitely the power and strength to do so. Joy and pleasure should be experienced, there should be no undue strain. Considerable attention must be paid to keeping up the rhythm. Remember that the rhythm is more important than the length of breath. Feel the rhythm throughout the whole body. Practice makes perfect. Patience and perseverance are needed.

Is mastery over the mechanics of breathing important?

Swami Niranjanananda: After learning to breathe consciously, it is necessary to learn to breathe completely, using the full capacity of the lungs. There are three basic mechanisms of breathing: i) abdominal or diaphragmatic, ii) thoracic or chest and, iii) clavicular or shoulder breathing. The normal breathing of an average person is a combination of thoracic and clavicular breathing. However, less effort is expended in diaphragmatic breathing to obtain the same quantity of air, so this type of breathing should be cultivated in daily life until it becomes a spontaneous habit. A complete revolution in the state of physical and mental wellbeing can be obtained by mastery of this technique. A combination of all three is known as full yogic breathing, which is a prerequisite of pranayama.

The breathing techniques alone, as a purely mechanical operation, create an appropriate effect on the body, mind and spirit. However, it has been observed that the effect of these techniques can be greatly amplified when they are applied with sensitivity and awareness of their subtle influences, and with a deeper understanding of the relationship between the body, energy and mind. The process becomes more efficient with awareness, and the inner knowledge begins to awaken.

ABDOMINAL, THORACIC AND CLAVICULAR BREATHING

What is abdominal breathing?

Swami Satyananda: Abdominal or diaphragmatic breathing is practised by enhancing the action of the diaphragm and minimizing the action of the ribcage. The diaphragm is a domed sheet of muscle that separates the lungs from the abdominal cavity and, when functioning correctly, promotes the most efficient type of breathing. It is the effect of the diaphragm rather than the diaphragm itself that is experienced as the stomach rises and falls, but sensitivity will come with practice. During inhalation the diaphragm moves downward, pushing the abdominal contents downward and outward. During exhalation the diaphragm moves upward and the abdominal contents move inward.

Movement of the diaphragm signifies that the lower lobes of the lungs are being used. The proper use of the diaphragm causes equal expansion of the alveoli, improves lymphatic drainage from basal parts of the lungs, massages the liver, stomach, intestines and other organs that lie immediately beneath it, exerts a positive effect on the cardiac functions and coronary supply, and improves oxygenation of the blood and circulation.

Abdominal breathing is the most natural and efficient way to breathe. However, due to tension, poor posture, restrictive clothing and lack of training, it is often forgotten.

Once this technique again becomes a part of daily life and correct breathing is restored, there will be a great improvement in the state of physical and mental wellbeing.

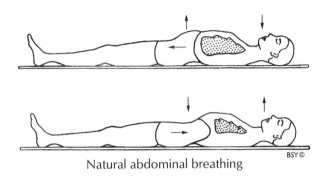

Natural abdominal breathing

BSY©

Why is abdominal breathing important?

Swami Niranjanananda: The diaphragm separates the lungs from the abdominal cavity. In normal breathing it hardly moves, but during deep breathing it extends downward into the abdomen on inhalation and upward on exhalation, promoting the most efficient type of breathing. Less effort is expended in diaphragmatic breathing to obtain the same quantity of air. Infants and small children use their diaphragms exclusively for breathing. Chest breathing occurs only later, after the bony structure of the chest matures.

Diaphragmatic breathing should be cultivated in daily life until it becomes a spontaneous habit. Nowadays, however, few have the ability to breathe with the abdomen due to tension, unhealthy habits, poor posture and tight clothing. A complete revolution in the state of physical and mental wellbeing can be obtained by mastery of this technique.

X-ray observations of diaphragmatic movement have shown that relaxed, pleasant thoughts and sensations increase its movement considerably while the breath becomes slower and deeper. Not only do relaxed thoughts allow muscle relaxation and greater diaphragmatic movement, but slow, relaxed breathing also calms the mind. Deep breathing has been observed to release endorphins into the bloodstream. The endorphins are potent brain chemicals which help one cope with pain and are part of the mechanism for dealing with and eliminating fear and anxiety.

What is thoracic breathing?

Swami Satyananda: Thoracic breathing uses the middle lobes of the lungs by expanding and contracting the ribcage. It expends more energy than abdominal breathing for the same quantity of air exchange. It is often associated with physical exercise and exertion, as well as stress and tension; when combined with abdominal breathing, it helps the body to obtain more oxygen. However, the tendency in many people is to continue this type of breathing, instead of abdominal breathing, long after the stressful situation has passed, creating bad breathing habits and continued tension.

What is clavicular breathing?

Swami Niranjanananda: Clavicular or shoulder breathing ventilates the upper lobes of the lungs. This type of breathing takes very little effort and is commonly preformed during sedentary activities. As a component of yogic breathing, it is the final stage of total ribcage expansion. It is performed after the thoracic inhalation has been completed in order to absorb a little more air into the lungs. In this type of breathing the upper ribs and collarbone are pulled upwards by the muscles on either side of the neck and throat. In daily life it occurs during such conditions as sobbing or an asthma attack.

Why does yoga teach thoracic and clavicular breathing?

Swami Niranjanananda: Thoracic breathing is a method of producing expansion and contraction of the ribcage. It is a less efficient type of breathing than abdominal breathing, but is required during increased physical activity, when a greater volume of air must be drawn into the lungs. In comparison with abdominal breathing, more muscular effort is required for the same quantity of air. Thoracic breathing is often associated with situations of mental stress and tension, as its function is to assist the lungs to gain more oxygen in a stressful situation. However, the tendency to continue this kind of breathing often remains long after the stressful situation has disappeared, creating bad breathing habits.

Thoracic breathing is inefficient because it brings the bulk of air into the middle lobes of the lungs, which are poorly supplied with blood. Detrimental effects include increased sympathetic nervous system dominance, increased heart rate and reduced carbon dioxide concentration in the blood.

Some people actually 'freeze' or immobilize the diaphragm and use the upper body to breathe in an attempt to hold back sexuality, fear, aggression and other powerful feelings. As these emotions are associated with mooladhara, swadhishthana and manipura chakras, stiffening the diaphragm serves to isolate the associated feelings in the lower body, pushing them out of awareness. However, intentional thoracic breathing in supportive settings can also be used to induce and release strong emotions and tension as a form of therapy.

Clavicular or shoulder breathing ventilates the upper lobes of the lungs, takes little effort and is commonly performed during sedentary activities. In daily life it occurs during such conditions as sobbing or an asthma attack. As a component of yogic breathing, it is the final stage of total ribcage expansion. It is performed after the thoracic inhalation has been completed in order to absorb a little more air into the lungs.

Thoracic and clavicular breathing should be practised for control over the full range of the breathing capacity. They are necessary in order to perform yogic breathing and certain pranayamas. There is no need to practise shoulder breathing on its own. It should only be practised long enough to be able to perform it efficiently during yogic breathing.

YOGIC BREATHING

What is yogic breathing?

Swami Niranjanananda: In yogic breathing, while inhaling, the lower lobes of the lungs are filled first, extending the diaphragm downward into the abdominal cavity and pushing the abdominal muscles outward. This is followed by thoracic breathing, which fills the middle lobes of the lungs, and creates an outward and upward movement of the ribcage. The inhalation is completed with clavicular breathing, which fills the upper lobes of the lungs, using the accessory muscles in the neck and shoulder girdle to further lift the ribcage.

The exhalation is the exact reverse of this process, with a combination of diaphragmatic and thoracic compression of the lungs to complete the expulsion of air. The lungs are stretched to maximum capacity on both inhalation and exhalation. All the stale air is expelled with each outgoing breath and the next inhalation brings fresh air to all the lobes of the lungs.

What is the purpose of yogic breathing?

Swami Niranjanananda: The purpose of yogic breathing is to gain control over the breathing process, correct poor breathing habits and increase the oxygen intake, when necessary. The practice of yogic breathing enables one to experience the complete range of each breathing mode. This bestows the numerous benefits of deep, fully-controlled breathing. As one exerts more control over the breathing process it becomes possible to control the finer details of the mental process.

Proficiency in yogic breathing means that all aspects of the breathing mechanism have come under the control of the conscious mind and can be controlled at will. This does not mean that yogic breathing should be practised at all times. During most pranayama techniques, yogic breathing is recommended. However, in pranayama it is not necessary to extend the breath into the clavicular region.

The combination of abdominal and thoracic breathing is optimum and produces a rhythmic wave of inhalation and exhalation.

What are the advantages of yogic breathing?
Swami Niranjanananda: In yogic breathing the lungs expand vertically as well as horizontally. The vertical expansion is promoted by increased diaphragmatic movement. During normal breathing the upward and downward movement of the diaphragm is approximately one centimetre, whereas in yogic breathing this movement may be as much as three to four centimetres. The sitting postures adopted during pranayama also promote greater expansion of the lungs in a vertical axis.

Normal, quiet and unconscious breathing moves half a litre (500 ml) of air into and out of the lungs (tidal volume). About a quarter of this volume (150 ml) is unused and occupies the spaces of the trachea and bronchi, which are merely air passages in which no exchange of gases occurs. Therefore, in normal breathing only a very small volume of fresh air actually enters the alveoli in the lungs with each breath.

In yogic breathing a much larger quantity of air reaches the lungs and inflates more alveolar tissue. During one full inhalation up to five litres of air may be taken in. Thus, more oxygen is made available for gas exchange with the blood. The increased vertical movement of the diaphragm also opens the alveoli of the lungs more evenly, particularly at the central, basal and apical areas of the lungs. Due to this even expansion, a greater expanse of alveolar membrane becomes available for gaseous exchange. The larger the surface area available, the more efficient is the gaseous exchange. In horizontal expansion, some alveoli may remain closed and collect secretions, causing them to become prone to disease. The possibility of this is reduced in yogic breathing.

MUDRAS AND BREATH

What is the relevance of mudras to pranayama?

Swami Niranjanananda: Within the pranamaya kosha, these mudras represent a linking of various circuits within the network of nadis, creating a flow of prana which has gross and subtle implications. Mudras induce a change in the pranic circulatory system; they activate the nadis, ensuring a smooth flow of prana and eliminating wastage of prana. Therefore, they are able to guide prana towards a specific organ, as intended by a specific mudra. The hand mudras in particular gradually rechannel the energy back into the system, others influence specific nadis and organs, and so on.

What is nasagra mudra?

Swami Niranjanananda: *Nasagra mudra* is one of the most common hand positions used in pranayama practice. It is sometimes known as nasikagra mudra. It is used to facilitate the smooth opening and closing of the nostrils required for

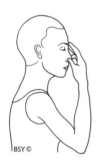

Nasagra mudra

alternate nostril breathing and therefore is of particular importance in nadi shodhana. Variations of the technique exist but the method generally taught is easy for beginners, as it is practical and efficient.

The right hand is used as it is more associated with giving on a pranic level, while the left is more associated with receiving. If, however, the right hand cannot be used for some reason, the left can be substituted.

What is hasta mudra pranayama?

Swami Niranjanananda: From the pranic point of view *mudras* represent a linkup of specific nadis in the body, in this case, in the fingers, by which prana is redirected to different areas.

Hasta mudra pranayama, the hand gesture breath, uses four specific hand positions known as *hasta* or hand mudras. These mudras are subtle techniques and their effects may not be immediately noticeable without awareness and sensitivity.

Hasta mudra pranayama uses hand mudras to ventilate the lower, middle and upper lobes of the lungs and influence other vital organs indirectly. The mudras used are: chin mudra for ventilation of the lower lobes of the lungs; chinmaya mudra for ventilation of the middle lobes of the lungs; aadi mudra for ventilation of the upper lobes of the lungs; and brahma mudra, for ventilation of the total lung capacity.

The pancha pranas are activated by these practices. They are also therapeutic, as they relieve disorders related to specific areas of the body. All four should be practised together in the sequence described, although for therapeutic purposes only the relevant practice need be applied.

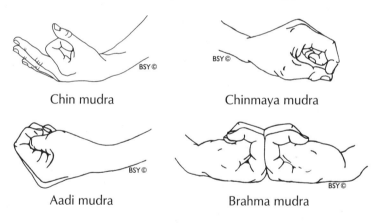

Chin mudra   Chinmaya mudra

Aadi mudra   Brahma mudra

How does chinmaya mudra affect the breath?

Swami Niranjanananda: Chinmaya mudra influences the prana and stimulates movement in the thoracic area creating subtle expansion of the breath in the middle lobes of the lungs. The acupuncture meridian points concerned here affect respiration.

How does aadi mudra affect the breath?

Swami Niranjanananda: When held, aadi mudra influences the breathing in the upper lobes of the lungs. While holding aadi mudra one should observe the effect on the upper chest region and clavicles.

What is the effect of brahma mudra on the breath?

Swami Niranjanananda: Brahma mudra helps to stimulate full yogic breathing, i.e. using the abdomen, chest and clavicles for each respiration. The knuckles, being pressed together, connect all the hand meridians. The tips of the fingers form another circuit as they touch the palm.

What are the prana vayu mudras?

Swami Niranjanananda: The five different kinds of prana vayu are represented and invoked by hand mudras. When performing these mudras, it does not mean that particular vayu is automatically felt surging through its normally specified location in the body, but on a subtle or pranic level that particular energy will be stimulated. While dealing with prana and its subtleties, one should have knowledge of these mudras, until finally a deeper awareness dawns of the vital energies, and of those same energies pervading the cosmos.

These mudras may be used with any pranayama or pre-pranayama practice when alternate nostril breathing with nasikagra mudra is not used.

The prana vayu mudras are:

Prana mudra: The tip of the thumb (fire), middle finger (space) and ring finger (earth) are placed together. The mantra used with this mudra is *Om Pranaya Swaha*. Prana vayu is located in the chest area.

Apana mudra: The tip of the thumb, index (air) and middle fingers are placed together. The mantra is *Om Apanaya Swaha*. Apana vayu is located in the pelvic area.

Samana mudra: The tip of the thumb, little finger (water) and ring finger are placed together. The mantra used is *Om Samanaya Swaha*. Samana vayu is located in the abdomen.

Udana mudra: The tip of the thumb, index and little fingers are placed together. The mantra is *Om Udanaya Swaha*. Udana vayu is located in the arms, legs, neck and head.

Vyana mudra: The tip of the thumb, index, middle, ring and little fingers are placed together. Its mantra is *Om Vyanaya Swaha*. Vyana vayu permeates the whole body.

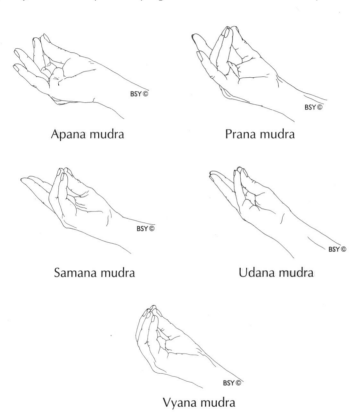

Apana mudra   Prana mudra

Samana mudra   Udana mudra

Vyana mudra

3

Benefits and Effects of Pranayama

EFFECTS ON BODY AND MIND

What are the outer signs and inner experiences of those who practise pranayama?

Swami Sivananda: By the practice of pranayama one can become a veritable god. Certain symptoms manifest when the nadis are purified. He who practises pranayama will have good appetite, cheerfulness, handsome figure, good strength, courage, enthusiasm, a high standard of health, vigour and vitality and good concentration of mind. The body becomes light, slender and healthy. There is lustre in the face and the eyes sparkle like diamonds. One's voice becomes sweet and melodious. In *Hatharatnavali* (3:95) it is written:

> *Yadaa tu naadeeshuddhih syaattadaa chihnaani baahyatah;*
> *Kaayasya krishataa kaantistathaa jaayeta nishchitam.*

When the nadis are purified, there are external signs. Slimness of the body and lustre are certain.

The breath can be retained for a long time. The inner anahata sounds are distinctly heard. The digestive fire is strong, perfect health is enjoyed, and one is cheerful and happy. This is also described in *Hatharatnavali* (3:96):

Yatheshtam dhaaranam vaayoranalasya pradeepanam;
Naadaabhivyaktiraarogyam jaayate naadishodhanaat.

By purifying the nadis one is able to retain the breath
with ease; the gastric fire is increased and experience of
(internally aroused) sound and good health are secured.

Rajas and tamas are destroyed. The mind is prepared for
dharana and dhyana. Steady practise of pranayama arouses
the inner spiritual force and brings ecstatic joy, spiritual light
and peace of mind. A yogi attains longevity by the practice
of pranayama.

**How does pranayama help one tune in to subtle forces
within the body and mind?**

Swami Niranjanananda: The rhythms of the breath relate to
the brain rhythms, heartbeat, muscle tension, mental and
emotional rhythms, hormonal and enzymatic rhythms, sleep
and wakefulness, all with varying frequencies and intensities.
These rhythms also take place within the external rhythms
of day and night, seasons, years and planetary influences.
Pranayama leads to the awareness of a rhythmic force
within the body and mind. When one becomes aware of
the body's vital cycles, they begin to work more optimally.
Simultaneously, the mind can be trained to control these
forces, thereby opening up areas of consciousness which are
beyond the normal awareness and control.

**Why is pranayama recommended for the management of
disease?**

Swami Niranjanananda: *Prana* means life force, and *ayama*
signifies regulation or control. Thus *pranayama* means
regulating the life force. Sages have linked this life force with
the breath in a gross form. Every living being breathes, and
through the medium of the breath the flow of prana and
life in the body takes place. If one stops inhaling, the lack of
prana in the body is felt, discomfort and unrest prevail and
if one is forced to keep on holding the breath, death finally

comes. For this reason the sages have linked the breath with the life force. According to them, physical health can be gained by controlling prana shakti through the practices of pranayama, thus sustaining the body. In this context it is written in *Gheranda Samhita* (5:1):

Athaatah sampravakshyaami praanaayaamasya sadvidhim;
Yasya saadhanamaatrena devatulyo bhavennarah.

Now I shall explain the technique of pranayama, by the mere practice of which a human being becomes like a god (a deva).

Sage Gheranda has compared the human body to a *deva sharira*, the body of a divine being or god, which is pure, clean, light, free from disease and luminous. He has taught pranayama with the intention of achieving such a divine body. This indicates that many problems can be eliminated by pranayama practice. Pranayama is the basis of the yogic management of disease. Diseases can be divided into three groups.

The first group is psychosomatic. Disorders related to this group begin with the mind, feelings and thinking. Worries and disturbances like anger, jealousy and hatred, which originate in the mind, influence the body and its internal activities, and various symptoms begin to arise.

The second group consists of disorders due to pranic blockages. When there are obstructions in the flow of prana, and the breathing process is disturbed, ailments related to breathing and blood pressure develop.

The third group originates externally, the external environment affects the body. Diseases like malaria, cholera and many others are caused by microorganisms attacking the body; other causes are pollution and irregular and uncontrolled eating.

Yoga recognizes these three most common causes of disease. There are also many other minor causes and ailments which can be managed with yogic techniques.

Sage Gheranda prescribes pranayama for the treatment of all diseases linked with the breathing system and the flow of prana. In the present era, research has proved that a large number of psychosomatic, somopsychic diseases and mental imbalances like distress and worry can be removed by pranayama.

What are the benefits of pranayama for the body's physical systems?

Swami Niranjanananda: The benefits of consistent pranayama practice for the systems of the body are many. The functioning of the respiratory, circulatory, digestive, excretory, endocrine and nervous systems becomes healthier, stronger and more efficient in those who practise pranayama regularly.

Pranayama exercises the muscles of respiration and the lungs through the processes of deep, rapid or slow breathing. This strengthens the respiratory muscles and makes the lungs more elastic, resulting in a healthier process of respiration. The training given to the respiratory organs and muscles during the pranayama practice prepares them to work efficiently throughout the day. With more efficient respiratory apparatus, a larger quantity of oxygen is absorbed than otherwise.

Similar benefits are received by the organs of digestion, absorption and elimination. The stomach, pancreas, liver, bowels and kidneys are all exercised in pranayama through the massage given by the accentuated movement of the diaphragm and abdominal muscles. All the associated muscles and nerves are toned up and rendered healthier.

Many studies have verified that pranayama is extremely beneficial for the heart. The practices minimize the stress put on the cardiac system by day-to-day life. Breathing with slow, deep and long breaths gives rest to the heart. During the practices of pranayama, the muscles of the heart are gently massaged, allowing for good circulation. In bhastrika and kapalbhati, vibrations spread to the entire circulatory system, including the veins, arteries and capillaries, making them function more efficiently. Many heart conditions can be managed through pranayama.

Pranayama harmonizes, purifies and neutralizes the secretions of the endocrine glands and thereby influences thought and behaviour. The overall health of the endocrine system is largely dependent on the quality of the blood and its distribution to the glands. The richer and more liberal blood supply brought to the endocrine glands by pranayama, particularly the vitalizing practices, enhances their functioning, and the regulated breathing helps balance the system.

The brain, spinal cord, cranial and spinal nerves benefit from the richer and more liberal blood supply. The inclusion of bandhas gives peripheral stimulus to the different nerve plexuses situated in the abdomen and thorax.

When one breathes slowly, deeply and in a systematic and coordinated manner, the neurons fire more rhythmically and the electrical interactions between the brain centres become more regulated. This means that wild fluctuations of the brainwaves are streamlined and there is balance between the two hemispheres of the brain. There are longer alpha waves and a reduction of beta waves. Alpha waves bring harmony to the brain as well as the coronary, respiratory and circulatory systems. People suffering from high blood pressure are benefited by influencing the alpha wave behaviour of the brain. By practising pranayama systematically for a few years, a gradual transformation is brought about in the structure of the nervous system. Ultimately, there comes a moment when one closes the eyes, goes in and achieves meditation.

Does pranayama increase physical and mental vitality?

Swami Niranjanananda: Through a physical process of releasing tension, the practice of asana removes blockages so that energy circulates efficiently through the system. But there may be a lack of energy, in which case it can be built up with the help of pranayama. The breath plays an important role in life without one's knowledge. A person breathes from the time of birth and will continue breathing until the time of death, but the experience of the breath tends to be limited to the external.

The way one breathes affects the level of vitality. Via pranayama the breath can be used to raise the vitality. The breath is linked with the state of one's nervous system. By breathing in slowly and deeply the state of the nervous system can be altered and the brain can be influenced. The activity of the brain can be altered in terms of the brainwaves, and simultaneously the mind is influenced. Yoga says that the breath is linked with prana, and *prana* means vital force, vital energy. Prana is the energy which is directly related with life and which is expanded with the practices of pranayama.

The practices connect the individual with the source of energy so that one's physical and mental energies do not become depleted. This brings about continuous alertness and a sense of wellbeing, dynamism and vitality. The purpose of pranayama is not to learn how to breathe properly but to awaken the inherent energy, the power or prana, within.

The process of energization through pranayama can be understood from another perspective. Pranayama creates static electricity in the body which helps to recharge the positive ions breathed in from the environment and convert them into negative ions. The effect is the same as that created by rain and thunderstorms. Hot and sultry weather makes one feel lethargic, but the air becomes fresh and clean with rain, and one feels energized and dynamic. Rain and thunderstorms charge the positive ions in the environment and convert them into negative ions. Similarly, pranayama generates static electricity in the body in minute quantities and there is a feeling of improved energy and dynamism.

How does pranayama help yogis to live in extreme conditions?

Swami Satyananda: In the Himalayas, and other places of the world, there are many mahatmas, rishis and sannyasins who live extremely austere lives. They are able to maintain themselves by preserving and increasing the *prana shakti*, or life force, in their physical body. Through intense practice of raja yoga, hatha yoga and dhyana yoga, they are able to completely change the nature and chemical structure of the body so as to withstand these extreme conditions.

What is the effect of pranayama on the mind?

Swami Sivananda: If the breath is unsteady, the mind is unsteady. If the breath is steady and calm, the mind is steady and calm. There is no purificatory action greater than pranayama. Pranayama gives purity, and the light of knowledge shines. The karma of the yogi, which covers up the light and binds him to repeated births, is attenuated by the practice of pranayama, and eventually is destroyed. Manu[1] says, 'Let the defect be burnt up by pranayama.' In the *Yoga Sutras* (2:53) Sage Pantanjali says, 'By the practice of pranayama the mind becomes fit for concentration.'

The mind can concentrate once these defects of karma have been removed. The mind will become quite steady, like the flame in a windless place, as the disturbing energy has been removed. When the prana moves in *akasha tattwa*, the ether principle, the breathing lessens. At this time it is easy to stop the breath. The velocity of the mind is slowly reduced by pranayama.

Dispassion arises. The student becomes so perfected in brahmacharya that his mind will not be shaken even if a celestial nymph tries to embrace him. His appetite becomes keen, the nadis are purified and tossing of the mind is removed as it becomes one-pointed. Rajas and tamas are destroyed. The mind is prepared for concentration, *dharana*,

---

[1] Manu: the first law-giver, the father of the human race.

and meditation, *dhyana*. Steady practice arouses inner spiritual light, happiness and peace of mind.

Why is pranayama good for calming the mind and senses?
Swami Sivananda: Some yogis practise *pooraka*, inhalation, some yogis practise *rechaka*, exhalation, and some yogis practise *kumbhaka*, retention of breath. The five sub-pranas and the other pranas are merged in the chief prana, *mukhya prana*, by the practice of pranayama. When the prana is controlled, the mind stops its wanderings and becomes steady, and the senses are thinned out and merged in the prana. It is through the vibration of prana that the activities of the mind and the senses are kept up. If the prana is controlled, the mind, intellect and senses cease to function. This pratyahara is described in the *Bhagavad Gita* (4:29):

Apaane juhvati praanam praane'paanam tathaapare;
Praanapaanagati ruddhvaa praanaayaamaparaayanaah.

Others offer as sacrifice the outgoing breath in the incoming, and the incoming in the outgoing, restraining the course of the outgoing and the incoming breaths, solely absorbed in the restraint of the breath.

How can pranayama help one to relax?
Swami Satyananda: Commonly, relaxation means an easy chair, a cup of tea or coffee, and a television, "Oh, I am relaxing now". No! In yoga, relaxation means freeing the whole system from tension – not only the physical body, but also the conscious and subconscious mind. Sometimes when the physical body is resting, the mind is not. Sometimes the conscious mind is relaxing but the subconscious mind is not.

If tranquillizers are taken, the conscious mind and body may be relaxed, but deep rooted worrying still goes on. Pranayama can be used effectively to bring about total relaxation and emotional integration, because in this system perpetual awareness is maintained while bringing the mind down to deeper levels of the subconscious.

Why is the ratio of 1:2 so important in pranayama?

Swami Satyananda: With the practice of pranayama, more oxygen may be inhaled but that is not the important point. If oxygen alone is the purpose, then deep breathing would be sufficient. In pranayama, inhalation and exhalation are practised in the ratio of 1:2, as this ratio is most beneficial for the heart. The pulse rate shows that with inspiration the heart rate speeds up, whereas with expiration it slows down. Therefore, when the ratio of 1:2 is used, there is an overall effect of relaxation of the coronary muscles, but without any reduction in the supply of oxygen to the brain and body tissues. If a ratio of 1:4 is practised, however, the effect of relaxation is cancelled because the brain accelerates the heart rate in reaction to a decreased supply of oxygen in the blood.

How can pranayama be used to balance the nervous system?

Swami Niranjanananda: When someone who is feeling hyperactive practices bhramari or nadi shodhana pranayama, within a few minutes they start to experience tranquillity in the mind and brain. On the other hand, if a person is depressed, and his awareness, his energy, is centred inside and he is unable to come out of the state of depression, then by practising bhastrika or kapalbhati pranayama, that concentrated state of energy which is drawing the mind inwards, will be rectified.

This change in the realm of *chitta*, mind, and *prana*, dynamic energy, takes place during the practices of pranayama and pratyahara, as certain psychic centres situated within the body are stimulated by the practices. For example, if a person who is hyperactive, tense or dissipated begins to practise pranayama, the controlled inhalations and exhalations begin to relax and control the activity of the nervous system. With the regulation of the nervous system in the body, the automatic activities, such as the heartbeat and blood pressure, come into balance.

This state of physical balance will gradually influence cerebral activity, lower the high beta frequency, and induce the alpha state, in which feelings of relaxation and ease develop. The dissipated mind slowly comes to a state of relaxation, focusing at a point. The balancing energy of ida then begins to flow in the system, and the hyperactivity slowly reduces in intensity, as the person becomes centred. Through the pranayama, the body has been worked on at the level of the nervous system, at the level of the autonomic functions, at the level of the brain, and then gradually, at the level of external perceptions, centring both them and the mind.

Why is pranayama said to be like mental shankhaprakshalana?

Swami Satyananda: During the practice of pranayama, purging takes place. If one starts practising bhastrika pranayama daily, after a few days, crazy ideas might start coming into the mind and there will be many funny thoughts and dreams. Some people feel frightened when this happens. They go to a swami and say, "Since I started practising pranayama, I've been getting crazy ideas." The swami answers, "Look here, shankhaprakshalana is going on." In yoga this is called cleaning of the mind – *chitta shuddhi*.

How can basic pranayama equip us to face and understand life?

Swami Satyananda: In order to face and understand life, in order to be unaffected by life, one has to change the structure and the quality of one's mind. If a person practises deep breathing, or vigorous breathing, or even wild breathing for half an hour and then lies down on the floor, they will feel light, they may even feel great bliss for half an hour, maybe one hour, maybe half a day.

But the moment any mental problem arises, all that has been gained, all that has been experienced by that wild breathing will be finished, because the changes that it produced were only in the co-ordination or mutual reaction of the nervous system. The change did not take place in the consciousness, in the philosophy, in the capacity to understand the events of life.

Therefore, side by side with bhastrika, with deep breathing, with vigorous or even with wild breathing, one must continue with spiritual practices. This is called restructuring of the mind. Only then will the delight remain perennial.

What is the effect of pranayama on the link between prana and the mind?

Swami Satyananda: Yoga says that the life force controls the mind, and the mind controls the life force. In yoga, the life force is called prana. This term prana refers to the individual life force as well as the cosmic life force. Prana is not the breath that is inhaled or the oxygen by which one lives. The life force is a creative force, which is responsible for existence and for evolution. When there is disturbance in the life force, there is disturbance in the mind. In yoga, there are two clear concepts: the total life force, which is called macrocosmic life, and the individual life force, known as microcosmic life. In the same way there is macrocosmic mind and microcosmic mind. So, if one wants to control the mind, one must learn to control the prana. Or if one wants to control the pranic force, then first the mind should be controlled.

How to control the prana? The pranas should be controlled through the practice of pranayama, which is linked through this body to the cosmic prana. Just as a person has an electromagnetic field through which energy flows, in the same way, the body has a pranic field. Not only inside but also outside the body, there is a pranic field linking each person with that cosmic pranic field.

Here is an example to illustrate the point. If the radio is switched on and tuned to certain frequencies, it will connect with the BBC, Voice of America or another station.

Whichever frequencies are tuned into, the connection is immediate, because there is a link. In the same way, the pranic field, the life field in this physical body, is linked with the cosmic prana, with the total pranic force. In order to communicate with the higher field of prana, one must first purify one's individual pranic force through yoga practices.

How can mental stability be attained?

Swami Satyananda: Yoga says that the prana, the breath and the mind are interrelated. When the mind is disturbed, the pranas are also disturbed. When the pranas are disquiet the mind also becomes disquiet. When one concentrates on the breath, the mind becomes concentrated. When one concentrates on the mind, the pranas become quiet. Just as electricity, light and heat are inseparable, the prana and the mind are inseparable.

Pranayama revitalizes and gives one the energy needed to manage daily problems and overcome all obstacles on the journey through life. During moments of anxiety, insecurity, fear and passion, instead of fighting with the mind through the intellect, take the help of pranayama to stabilize the mind. It is the way to mental peace, physical health, revitalization and longevity.

Pranayama brings new levels of awareness by stopping or restraining distractions of the mind. In other words, it is the continual conflict within the mind that prevents us from experiencing higher states or dimensions of awareness. Pranayama practices reduce thoughts, mental conflicts etc., to a minimum and can even stop the mind processes completely. This restraint of mental activities allows one to know higher levels of existence.

Here is an analogy. If one stands in a room and looks at the sun through a dirty window then the rays of the sun cannot be seen or felt in their full purity. If the window is cleaned then the sun can be experienced in its true glory. The mind in its normal state is the dirty window. Pranayama cleans the mind and allows the consciousness to shine

71

through unobstructed. It becomes obvious that pranayama means far more than breath control.

What is the effect of pranayama on thought processes and the mental state?

Swami Satyananda: An aspirant of pranayama need not worry about the mind, the mind does not exist for him. For the aspirant of pranayama, the wild mind, this dirty and foul mind does not exist, because as the practice of pranayama goes on, the pranic force keeps pushing into the dark areas of consciousness and life, and as this happens, the mind is evaporating.

The individual mind is a concept; there is no individual mind. There is no thought process. Thoughts are impressions. Reading something creates an impression. One becomes aware of impressions stage by stage, and so it seems that they are moving. But thoughts don't move – they don't travel into the past, present and future, they are just there, that's all.

When the structure of the physical is changed, the mental substance automatically undergoes a change. The mind is a further manifestation of the body, and when the mind is influenced, the spirit is also influenced. Body, mind and spirit are not 'the trinity'- they are the unity, one. This is the understanding behind the practices of pranayama and hatha yoga.

Can pranayama help control our emotional, mental and intellectual expressions?

Swami Niranjanananda: The breath is intimately related to the states of emotion and intellect. The breath is taken for granted and so there is a failure to understand that by harmonizing the breathing patterns, one's emotions, mind and intellect can also be influenced and altered.

Everyone knows that when they feel afraid or angry the breathing becomes rapid and shallow. Conversely, when one is relaxed and tension-free, the breath becomes slow and deep. The breath controls certain aspects of the nervous system, the activity of the brain, and emotional and intellectual expression. The practice of pranayama gives voluntary control over the intellectual and emotional patterns and activities.

Scientists are investigating the relationship between breath and mind, because a relationship is definitely there. By observing one's breath-the length, the speed etc.,-the state of one's emotions and intellect can be determined. The activity of the brain and what type of experiences one is having can be known by simply observing it. Moods can be altered and controlled – the moods of the emotions and the moods of the intellect.

When there is a lot of dissipation and distraction and it is not possible to focus the mind, if breath observation is practised for just a few minutes, the mind suddenly becomes one-pointed. When a person is tense, or angry, if by chance they happen to observe the breath, they will observe that it is coming out quickly, in short spurts. This is shallow or upper thoracic breathing. On the other hand, during relaxation, the breathing becomes slow and deep.

How does breath retention affect the pranic and mental bodies?

Swami Niranjanananda: Many different types of investigations have proved that there is a relationship between breath and mind. Studies have also gone further, showing that there is a definite relationship between the consciousness and the breath at the time of inhalation and exhalation, and at the time of internal and external breath retention.

During inhalation, resistance is built up: physiologically, resistance is built up in the nervous, muscular and circulatory systems, and in the brain. There is a state of alertness. During exhalation, this resistance slowly dissipates, leaving the experience of relaxation. When the breath is held in, there is expansion of the pranic field within the body and the electrical emissions from the body. A form of this can be seen in Kirlian photography.

After internal retention, the electromagnetic field of the body greatly increases, and after exhalation the same field contracts. During pranayama, therefore, the pranamaya kosha undergoes the same experience of expansion and contraction as the physical body.

In the mind one also creates and reduces resistance. How can all this be monitored? There is one simple experiment which anyone can try. Fall into a rhythmic pattern of breathing and ask someone to say a sentence at the time of inhalation and another sentence at the time of exhalation. The sentence repeated at the time of exhalation will be remembered more clearly, as due to the lower resistance of mind, intellect and body, it was absorbed more easily.

There are many systems developing around the world for accelerating learning. Yoga nidra, especially in the training of children, has been most effectively used by Swami Satyananda. He used the technique of telling the practitioner to observe the breath, the duration of retention, the duration of exhalation, the relaxation of the body and the state of mind, and then giving the instruction.

In yoga this technique is used a great deal for training the inner mind, the unconscious and the subconscious mind, because the mind as a whole is a form of energy related to pranamaya kosha. Of course, it has a separate identity, but the two are interlinked. Through pranamaya kosha the mind is influenced and through manomaya kosha the pranic field is influenced.

In brief, internal and external retention expand and contract the pranic field, causing an increase and decrease in mental or intellectual resistance. If pranayama is incorporated before yoga nidra, it lowers the emotional resistance, and in this way the mind can be reprogrammed more effectively.

What are the outcomes of correct and incorrect practice of pranayama?

Swami Satyananda: Regular, ongoing and correct practice of pranayama activates sushumna nadi. Normally the energy in the nadis fluctuates from ida to pingala, but when the energy is equally balanced in both they cease to function and the energy rises through sushumna. In *Hatha Yoga Pradipika* (2:41) it is said:

Vidhivatpraanasamyaamairnaadeechakre vishodhite;
Sushumnaavadanam bhittva sukhaadvishati maarutah.

By systematically restraining the prana, the nadis and chakras are purified. Thus, the prana bursts open the doorway to sushumna and easily enters it.

If pranayama is practised incorrectly, it could create an imbalance but nothing disastrous will happen. If done specifically as instructed by the guru, it will definitely arouse kundalini in this lifetime. When pranayama is done correctly, it is like sowing potent seeds in fertile soil. When practised incorrectly, it is like planting small stones in the soil, believing them to be seeds and expecting plants to grow. No matter how much you water the stones they will never develop into plants.

Can the practices of pranayama cause disturbing effects?
Swami Satyananda: By practising pranayama correctly, the mind is automatically conquered. But the effects of pranayama are not always simple to manage. Pranayama may create extra heat in the body, awaken various centres in the brain and possibly affect the production of sperm and testosterone. It can also bring down the temperature of the inner body and the rate of respiration, and change the brainwave patterns. When these changes take place, a practitioner who is not adequately prepared may not be able to handle it. In *Hatharatnavali* (3:92) a warning is given:

Praanaayaamena yuktena sarvarogakshayo bhavet;
Ayuktaabhyaasayogena sarvarogasamudbhavah.

By proper practice of pranayama, all diseases are annihilated. Improper practice of pranayama, on the other hand, gives rise to all sorts of diseases.

However, the experiences that are described in the hatha yoga books are about the high or highest stage of pranayama. Therefore, the whole thing must be correctly understood. When pranayama is practised for half an hour these things won't take place. Neither itching nor perspiration will take place. If one practises pranayama for three to five hours, these symptoms will manifest, but they have nothing to do with the awakening of kundalini: they are symptoms that belong purely to the gross body.

How does pranayama remove the fear of death?

Swami Satyananda: Pranayama has a definite strengthening effect on the brain centres responsible for emotion and fear. In *Hatha Yoga Pradipika* (2:39–40), Swatmarama claims that fear of death can be eradicated through pranayama:

> *Brahmaadayo'pi tridashaah pavanaabhyaasatatparaah;*
> *Abhoovannantakabhayaattasmaatpavanamabhyaset.*

> *Yaavadbaddhomaruddehe yaavachchittam niraakulam;*
> *Yaavaddrishtirbhruvormadhye taavatkaalabhayam krutah.*

> Even Brahma and other gods in heaven devote themselves to practising pranayama, as it ends the fear of death. Thus, it must be practised. (39)

> As long as the breath is restrained in the body, the mind is devoid of thought and the gaze is centred between the eyebrows, why should there be fear of death? (40)

If the mind and prana are absorbed in the centre which is responsible for the experience of universal consciousness or *atma*, what can cause fear of death? When the individual soul or *jivatma* has merged into its source, experience is total, there is no individuality. Any thought of death cannot occur because 'you' do not exist. Fear only comes with the experience of duality. If one thinks there is something to lose, if there is a feeling of separation and no knowledge of unity, then there is fear of death.

76

Bodily processes are drastically altered when the mind and prana are totally absorbed during the experience of oneness. The breath is retained spontaneously, the eyeballs roll back as if gazing at the eyebrow centre, blood pressure, heart rate, pulse, metabolism and visceral functions are all altered. The body goes into a state of suspended animation and time and space do not exist in the mind. The body appears as if dead, but it isn't, as it has the capacity to regenerate prana. It is only suspended for a short while.

By practising breath retention and shambhavi mudra, and focusing the mind on a single point, the practitioner induces the state of complete absorption. If a superconscious state occurs, when one returns to mundane awareness, the thought of death has less significance. Whether the body is dead or alive is irrelevant to one who has realized the atma.

EFFECTS ON THE BRAIN

How does the extra prana generated by pranayama influence the brain?

Swami Satyananda: Under normal conditions a certain amount of prana is circulating, and this is responsible for the general level of health. However, pranayama is important because it enables one to consciously generate a higher voltage of prana and this greater quantity of prana can then be directed into the higher centres of the brain. In this way, pranayama brings an experience of a higher reality and dimension to its practitioner. It boosts the level of consciousness by activating and awakening the dormant centres and capacities of the evolving brain.

Does pranayama send prana to the brain?

Swami Satyananda: Pranayama is mainly concerned with the different levels of pranic energy. Prana is life. *Ayama* means dimensions. One dimension is the gross dimension, in which the breath goes into the lungs. But there are other dimensions, other spheres, where the prana can interpenetrate.

So where can this prana interpenetrate? Deep into the brain. It has been proved by science that when one breathes, the brain is breathing. Therefore, when one does pranayama, the brain is doing pranayama, not merely the lungs.

However, just practising a little pranayama doesn't mean one is sending a lot of prana to the brain. The process of supply and assimilation of prana into the brain is very complicated. The brain is a subtle instrument and it can only be enriched by the subtle form of prana and not the gross form. Therefore, when pranayama is practised, the prana has to be converted into a subtle force.

Deep breathing alone is not enough to stimulate prana. By breathing deeply, the respiratory system and blood circulation are stimulated, but the brain is least affected. However, scientific studies have shown that when pranayama is practised with concentration, the brainwaves undergo a significant change and the limbic system is positively influenced.

What effect does pranayama have on the brainwaves?

Swami Niranjanananda: Yogis did not have the concept of beta, alpha, theta and delta waves, but they had the concept of jagrat, swapna, sushupti and turiya, the four states of the mind. There is a distinct pattern of mental waves in all four states.

Jagrat describes full activity of the mind and brain, and in this full activity there is dissipation of energy. When beta waves are predominant in the brain, there is dissipation, activity and distraction. One is not relaxed, centred, balanced or focussed.

Swapna is literally translated as the state of dream, but in yoga it does not mean dream but a relaxed mind, one contained within itself. It is aware and alert. Swapna is the mind looking inwards. Jagrat describes the mind looking outwards, identifying name, form and idea, recognizing different things – this is *jagrat avastha*, the externally awake state. But in *swapna*, when the mind is looking inwards, it is seeing the internal experience, not the external objects. That experience is the same as the outer one of name, form, idea and quality, but the same thing that is perceived outside, is perceived inside. When everything is seen inside, the senses are focussed inwards and the experience of the mind is more passive. Tha alpha brainwave experience is this passive experience.

Then comes *nidra*, or sleep, where there is an absolute blank, deep relaxation, and theta waves; that state is called *sushupti avastha*. Beyond that, one can go deeper into that sate of relaxation and experience inner tranquillity. That is the *turiya* state. Intense concentration gives the delta state, the identification or experience of that deep relaxation which is leading one to harmony, balance and peace.

Pranayama activates the prana shakti in these mental sates and in the brain. Often people wake up in the morning, having slept for eight or ten hours, feeling physically and mentally exhausted. This indicates that sleep does not replenish prana shakti. Sleep only relaxes the body. The source of prana shakti is not sleep, it is the activation of ida and pingala nadis, and this activation is the purpose of pranayama.

Why is pranayama an important technique for controlling the mind?

Swami Satyananda: When one goes further into yoga, there comes a time when there must be some control of the mind, so that one can dive deeper inside. When a person tries to practise mantra or meditation, the fluctuating mental waves create a barrier between the meditator and the object which they are trying to focus the awareness on. So, how to control the mind?

Prana and mind are intricately linked. Fluctuation of one means fluctuation of the other. When either the mind or prana becomes balanced, the other is steadied. Hatha yoga says, control the prana and the mind is automatically controlled, whereas raja yoga says, control the mind and prana becomes controlled. These are two paths of yoga. In *Hatha Yoga Pradipika* (2:2) it is said:

> *Chale vaate chalam chittam nishchale nishchalam bhavet;*
> *Yogee sthaanutvamaapnoti tato vaayum nirodhayet.*

When prana moves, chitta (the mental force) moves. When prana is without movement, chitta is without movement. By this (steadiness of prana) the yogi attains steadiness and should thus restrain the vayu (air).

The mind is like a wild monkey, jumping here and there. Because of this inborn tendency it is difficult to hold it still. Hatha yoga says let the mind be, concentrate on the autonomic bodily functions and vital energy, and the mind will become quiet by itself. When the nervous impulses are steady and rhythmic, the brain functions are regulated and the brainwaves also become rhythmic.

The breathing process is directly connected to the brain and central nervous system, and is one of the most vital processes in the body. It is also connected with the hypothalamus, the brain centre which controls emotional responses. The hypothalamus is responsible for transforming perception into cognitive experience. Erratic breathing sends erratic impulses to this centre and thus creates disturbed responses.

There are also certain areas of the nasal mucous membrane which are connected to the visceral organs. When impulses coming from the nose are arhythmic, the visceral organs, particularly those connected to the coccygeal plexus, respond in the same manner, arhythmically. Being disturbed, these organs again send irregular impulses to the brain and cause more disharmony and imbalance. This cycle is continuous.

By becoming aware of the nature of the breath and by restraining it, the whole system is controlled. When the breath is retained, nervous impulses in different parts of the body are stopped, and brainwave patterns are harmonized. In pranayama, the duration of breath retention is gradually increased. The longer the breath is held, the greater the gap between nervous impulses and their responses in the brain. When retention is practised for a prolonged period, mental agitation is curtailed.

EFFECTS ON PRANA

What are the signs that the pranas are being awakened through pranayama?

Swami Sivananda: Dear child! Take sole refuge in pranayama. If the mind is solely turned towards pranayama, be interested in the practice of kumbhaka alone. The *Bhagavad Gita* says: "*Pranayama parayana* – solely absorbed in the control of breathing." Take due precaution at every step. The practice of kumbhaka produces tremendous heat in the body and thereby the kundalini is roused and sent upwards along the sushumna to the crown of the head.

In the first stage of pranayama there will be perspiration of the body. A tremor of the body will be experienced in the second stage. In the third stage, levitation manifests. In the final stage, the prana goes to the *brahmarandhara*, the hole of Brahma, at the top of the head. Sometimes the practitioner may jump like a frog. This is written in *Shiva Samhita* (3:40–41):

Svedah sanjaayate dehe yoginah prathamodyam;
Yadaa sanjaayate svedo mardanam kaarayetsidheeh
Anyathaa vigrahe dhaaturnashto bhavati yoginah.

Dviteeye hi bhavetkampo daarduree madhyame mataa;
Tato'dhikataraabhyaasaadgaganecharasaadhakah.

In the first stage of pranayama, the body of the yogi begins to perspire. When it perspires he should rub it well, otherwise the body of the yogi loses its dhatu (humours). (40)

81

In the second stage, there takes place the trembling of the body; in the third, the jumping about like a frog; and when the practice becomes greater, the adept walks in the air. (41)

What are the physical signs of pranic awakening?

Swami Satyananda: When the body and mind are purified, and the quantity of prana is increased, various physical symptoms manifest during pranayama. The body becomes hot due to peripheral vasodilatation. If it perspires irrespective of cool weather, pranic awakening has definitely taken place. It is possible for hot flushes to occur but excess heat is not necessarily noticed.

In the second stage, there may be quivering or sensations in the spine, or perhaps twitching of the hands, face and various other muscles. When the mind, body and breath become completely steady the practice is nearly perfect. The final stage is when the breath stops moving by itself.

Initially, when the pranic flow becomes intense, the peripheral parts of the body may vibrate. Impulses rush through the central nervous system and create itching or tingling sensations. The prana accumulates in different regions and may create strange sensations in the chest, abdomen, intestines or excretory organs, and sometimes whining sounds come from the lower intestines or excretory passage. In *Hatha Yoga Pradipika* (2:12) it is said:

Kaneeyasi bhavetsvedah kampo bhavati madhyama;
Uttame sthaanamaapnoti tato vaayum nibhandhayet.

At first there is perspiration, in the middle stage trembling, in the highest stage complete steadiness, and therefore the breath should be withheld.

What type of benefits does pranayama bring?

Swami Niranjanananda: The practice of pranayama is full of boons. The capacity to travel in space is attained. It provides bliss and alleviates every type of disease. It enhances the capacity for higher knowledge and inner vision. Through pranayama all types of physical, mental and spiritual benefits can be achieved. Both the subtle and gross bodies benefit. In *Gheranda Samhita* (5:57) the benefits of pranayama are described:

Praanaayaamaatkhecharatvam praanaayaamaadrujaam hatih;
Praanaayaamaachchhaktibodhah praanaayaamaanmanonmanee;
Aanando jaayate chitte praanaayaamee sukhee bhavet.

Through the practice of pranayama, travel in space, elimination of diseases and awakening of kundalini is achieved. Bliss manifests in the mind through pranayama and one becomes happy.

What effect does pranayama have on the body's prana?

Swami Satyananda: Through the practices of pranayama a certain amount of heat or creative force is generated in the entire body which influences the existing quantity of prana, just as if heat is produced in this room, the air will be heated. A certain amount of prana then makes its way through pingala nadi into ajna chakra. When sufficient heat is generated within the system, ajna chakra sends the message back to the base of kundalini and the actual awakening of the great prana takes place. This, in short, is the purpose of pranayama. This heating effect is described in *Hatharatnavali* (3:89):

Kaneeyasee bhavetsvedah kampo bhavati madhyama;
Uttishtheduttame praanarodhe padmaasanam muhuh.

Pranayama of a basic level generates sweat, that of an intermediate level, throbbing. And by pranayama practised in all its intensity, prana raises up (to sushumna). One should perform it in padmasana.

What is meant by purification of the pranic body through pranayama?

Swami Niranjanananda: At the pranic level, in their initial stages the practices of pranayama clear up the *nadis*, energy pathways in the body. The scriptures say there are over 72,000 nadis or pathways of prana in the pranic body and six main chakras. However, in the average individual, many of these pathways are blocked and the chakras release energy only partially. In other words, one's full potential is not used in terms of energy, mind and consciousness.

The negative conditions we experience, whether physical or mental, are the cause as well as the consequence of the blockages. The state of our nadis and chakras are defined by our *samskaras*, conditionings carried in seed form, as well as *purushartha*, self-effort and *anugraha*, grace. With the practice of pranayama, these pathways of energy are gradually freed so that prana moves through them smoothly.

At higher levels of practice, the direction of the pranic flows is influenced and a greater amount of energy is released from the chakras. As these processes are activated many new experiences unfold. Expert guidance is essential to steer the practitioner through these stages.

What effect does pranayama have on the distribution of prana in the body?

Swami Satyananda: The practice of pranayama forms the core of spiritual awakening. The practice of pranayama results in proper organisation of pranic energy in the body. With pranayama, prana is supplied to areas where it was scarce and any excess in other areas is balanced.

A certain quantity of prana exists in each human body. Prana flows in the body on a superficial level to maintain the body and its organs. The distribution of prana throughout the physical structure occurs via a system of thousands and thousands of subtle channels. Therefore, pranayama literally means supplying and balancing the pranic energy to different dimensions of the body.

Sometimes when one is relaxing, the prana is in the digestive system, or when one is eating, the prana is in the brain. When prana is needed in mooladhara or sahasrara, the body should be able to supply it. When one sits for meditation, excess prana is needed in the higher regions of the brain, and when one eats, more pranic energy is needed in the digestive system. Similarly, during the practice of yoga nidra or sleep, the prana should be distributed throughout the body.

What is the effect of blockages in the nadis?
Swami Niranjanananda: In pranayama practice, once the breath is controlled and harmonized, one moves into the dimension of prana. In that dimension one works with the nadis. Each nadi is a conductor of energy. If there is any block in these channels and energy does not flow, the corresponding organ of the body is affected. That is known as illness. The corresponding organ of the body becomes weak: it goes through the process of infirmity, weakness and old age at a faster rate than normal.

How can pranayama help one experience the subtle planes of existence?
Swami Satyananda: Pranayama is practised in order to extend the dimensions of prana. What are the dimensions of prana? Has prana many planes of existence? In which plane does prana flow? What happens if prana does not flow?

Once I had a dream which answered these questions for me. I was with my guru in a beautiful city with wide roads lined with electricity poles. I went into the buildings and found lights, telephones, televisions, everything – but there was no one in the city, and there was no electricity, the whole city was in complete darkness. I asked my guru, "That's a beautiful city, why is there no one here?" He replied, "They ask, what is the fun of being here when there is no electricity? When it is connected the whole city is illumined and everybody will like being here."

There are planes of existence which are in absolute darkness, much more beautiful and much more artistic than this. Those planes or areas of existence are in absolute darkness. How can one to bring them to light? How is one to penetrate them through experience? It is no use listening to talks or reading books, one must be able to penetrate those planes through experience, just as one experiences a dream. Even as one experiences sleep, so one should be able to experience those stages of consciousness.

Through the practice of pranayama it is possible to send the prana into those different dimensions. When the pranic energy is aroused, awakened through the practice of pranayama, and circulated through those dark areas of existence, then the purpose of pranayama is fulfilled.

What is the relationship between breath, prana and the lifespan?

Swami Niranjanananda: In order to maintain the vitality of the body, yogis advise the practices of pranayama. The word *pranayama* means to lengthen the prana. Yogis recognized that the prana which one breathes in is of low potency, only sufficient to make the body live for X number of minutes; if the potency of prana shakti can be lengthened and increased, expanding the dimension of prana, then by taking only a few breaths, one can be as active as if respiration was normal.

This result has been described in swara yoga which says that the slower one breathes, the longer one lives. If the breath can be deepened, one's lifespan will increase. If the breaths are short and shallow, the internal vital force is being used up and cannot be replenished by the air being breathed in. There is more wear and tear in the body and the lifespan is shortened.

Yogis have also observed different animals and noticed that animals which breathe fast have short lifespans, while animals that breathe slowly have longer lifespans. It has also been observed that on average a person breathes eleven times per minute, but a yogi who has perfected pranayama breathes only about three to five breaths per minute, and there is an increase in vitality.

86

What practices are needed in order to unite the flows of prana?

Swami Niranjanananda: In the dimension of prana, one works with nadis, the nadi system and the reversal of the pranic flows in the personality. Ideally, all the pranas should flow upwards, but in the manifest dimension different forms of prana flow in different directions. In order to aid the process of uniting the different flows of prana, along with the pranayamas, other practices known as mudras and bandhas are also used.

What is the relationship between cosmic energy, pranayama and meditation?

Swami Satyananda: In yoga, cosmic energy is known as prana. There is life energy in the whole atmosphere, but in addition to this there is an infinite quantity of cosmic energy. This energy is predominantly present in the five elements. Just as we say the source of protein is meat, eggs, nuts and soya beans, in the same way the five sources of prana are earth, water, fire, air and ether (space). But the best source of prana is the air, and that is why pranayama is such a powerful practice.

The breath which one takes inside is not pure prana; it is air with prana. Ultimately it is purified and separated into ordinary air and prana. This separation occurs during kumbhaka, and at the time of meditation these pranas are assimilated. Therefore, a hatha yogi who practises pranayama must also practise meditation in order to assimilate the separated prana. So this cosmic prana becomes a part of the individual prana through pranayama and meditation.

4

Pranayama Sadhana

GENERAL GUIDELINES

Why do many hatha yoga schools only teach asanas?

Swami Niranjanananda: Bihar School of Yoga was the first institute to teach pranayama. Previously there were no books on pranayama. Everybody used to say it was secret and had to be done under the guidance of the guru. But Swami Satyananda made it a rule that every yoga class must include asana, pranayama, a pratyahara technique like yoga nidra and one meditation practice. This made it a complete system to restore physical health and mental wellbeing.

What are the basic guidelines for practising pranayama?

Swami Sivananda: Observe brahmacharya and diet control. Pranayama should be practised when the stomach is empty. Practice must be regular. Do not take a bath immediately after the practice. Do not practise *kumbhaka*, retention of breath, in the beginning. Practise only slow and mild *pooraka*, inhalation, and *rechaka*, exhalation. Do not strain the breath beyond its capacity. The maximum benefits will be derived and the nadis will quickly be purified.

How important is a systematic approach to success in pranayama?

Swami Sivananda: Be regular and systematic in practising pranayama. Do not miss even a single day, unless seriously ailing from some disease. Regularity in the practice is absolutely necessary if one wants to realize the maximum benefits of pranayama. Those who practise by fits and starts will not derive much benefit. Generally people practise for two months with great enthusiasm and then leave the practice. This is a sad mistake. Avoid as much as possible too much talking, eating, sleeping, mixing with friends and all exertion.

Commence mild pranayama with inhalation and exhalation for one month. Pranayama can also be practised while walking. This suits some busy people who do not have much time to spare. Practise the various prescribed exercises one by one, step by step. Never be in a hurry. Never go beyond capacity. Do not take up a higher exercise before completely mastering the previous one. This is the master key to success in pranayama.

There is no use jumping from one pranayama to another every day. One must have a particular pranayama for daily practice which is improved to an advanced stage. Other pranayamas may be used for occasional practice along with the daily pranayama. Have pranayamas such as bhastrika, kapalbhati, and nadi shodhana for daily practice, and pranayamas such as sheetali and sheetkari for occasional use. In *Hatharatnavali* (3:94) the importance of regulated practice is emphasized:

Yuktam yuktam tyajedvaayum yuktam yuktam cha poorayet;
Yuktam yuktam cha badhneeyaat evam siddhimavaapnuyaat.

One should exhale, retain and inhale in a regulated manner and should in this way attain success in pranayama.

There should be a feeling of joy and exhilaration when the pranayama is over, but do not expect results after doing

89

pranayama for two or three minutes for a few days only. Practice must be for at least fifteen minutes daily for several months before fruits of the pranayama will be experienced.

What rules and regulations should be observed when practising pranayama?
Swami Satyananda: In the traditional texts there are innumerable rules and regulations pertaining to pranayama. The main points are to exercise moderation, balance and common sense with regard to inner and outer thinking and living. In *Hatha Yoga Pradipika* (2:1) it is said:

> *Athaasane dridhe yogee vashee hitamitaashanah;*
> *Guroopadishtamaarge praanaayaamaansamabhyaset.*

> Thus, being established in asana and having control (of the body), taking a balanced diet, pranayama should be practised according to the instructions of the guru.

When the body is regulated by asana and moderate diet, a sadhaka should begin the next stage of hatha yoga, which is pranayama. Pranayama is more than simple breathing exercises, and it must be practised systematically and under proper guidance according to the instructions of the guru.

Pranayama is practised in order to understand and control the pranic process in the body. Breathing is a direct means of absorbing prana and the manner in which one breathes sets off pranic vibrations which influence the entire being. Diet control is specified along with the practice of pranayama. Eating is a direct means of pranic absorption, affecting the body, mind and pranic vibrations.

Pranayama should not be practised during illness and the contra-indications given for individual practices should always be carefully observed. Pranayama must be practised on an empty stomach and with empty bowels. One should not even take tea before practising.

It is important to practise neti kriya before practising pranayama. This cleanses the nasal passages. Those who

90

suffer from hyperacidity, should practise kunjal kriya, which cleanses the stomach.

Pranayama should be practised in a firm posture like siddhasana, padmasana, sukhasana or vajrasana. Pranayama should not be practised without first performing yoga postures or *asanas*.

But the most important rule is, do not practice pranayama just from books, have a teacher. For those who wish to seriously take up the advanced practices of pranayama, the guidance of a guru or competent teacher is essential.

What are the essential rules for pranayama practice?

Swami Niranjanananda: In order to practise pranayama, it is essential to follow certain rules. Intense pranayama sadhana cannot be practised under normal conditions: a separate place, separate food and separate guidelines are required. Normally, the guidelines advocated for the practice of pranayama are simply to keep the body and mind healthy and balanced, and to focus the mind. To gain more benefits, however, strict rules must be observed. The basic guidelines are given in *Gheranda Samhita* (5:2):

> *Aadau sthaanam tathaa kaalam mitaahaaram tathaaparam;*
> *Naadeeshuddhim tatah pashchaatpraanaayaamam cha saadhayet.*

> First select the place and time, eat moderately and purify the nadis. After this, pranayama should be practised.

Aadau sthaanam, firstly a place for the practice of pranayama should be chosen. *Tathaa kaalam*, after this a time should be fixed. The practices of pranayama should only be done at the correct time and place. *Mitaahaaram tathaaparam*, then moderate food should be organized. *Naadeeshuddhim tatah pashchaatpraanaayaamam cha saadhayet*, when the place, time and food have been arranged, then before commencing pranayama, the nadis should be purified.

Generally speaking, the rules pertaining to the place and time prescribed for yoga practice are well known.

1. Pranayama should be practised during brahmamuhurta, not during the daytime. *Brahmamuhurta* means the two hours around dawn, between 4 and 6 am, best suited to yoga sadhana.
2. When the air is mild, slow and cool, not too cold and not too hot, pranayama should be practised.
3. Pranayama should never be practised in a closed room. Keep the windows and doors open to ensure that pure air can enter. However, the place should not be so airy or windy that the blast of the wind can be felt inside the room.
4. If the air is slightly cool or chilly, cover the body with a shawl or wear a vest. The body should not be allowed to come into direct contact with cold air. The practice of pranayama is also prohibited if there is sweating due to intense heat.

What is the correct approach to developing the practices of pranayama?

Swami Niranjanananda: In pranayama, lung capacity and flexibility of the muscles used in breathing should be developed gradually. During pranayama, one should never be left without air. Attention must be paid to what is happening in the body, and how it reacts to certain breathing techniques, so as to estimate its current limits. The purpose of all physical yogic techniques is to create balance and harmony in the body, not stress. If one is left without air, it creates stress in the body. This point is made in *Hatharatnavali* (3:91):

> *Yathaa simho gajo vyaaghro bhavedvashyah shanaih shanaih;*
> *Tathaiva sevito vaayuranyathaa hanti saadhakah.*

> Just as a lion, an elephant or a tiger is tamed by degrees, similarly respiration is to be brought under control gradually; otherwise it would harm the aspirant.

Why is it important to practise pranayama precisely and systematically?

Swami Satyananda: When pranayama is performed correctly and systematically, in the proper proportion, and in a steady sitting position, prana is channelled into the higher brain centres which are responsible for greater psychic capacity. Nothing can ever be attained by just inhaling and exhaling in any fashion or in the usual way. In *Hatha Yoga Pradipika* (2:18) it is said:

Yuktam yuktam tyajedvaayum yuktam yuktam cha poorayet;
Yuktam yuktam cha bandheeyaadevam siddhimavaapnuyaat.

The vayu should skilfully be inhaled, exhaled and retained so that perfection or siddhi is attained.

The word *yuktam* is used repeatedly in this verse to emphasize the necessity of precision. Just as an engineer who works with precision becomes perfect in his profession, in the same way, the sadhaka who practises pranayama precisely and systematically develops physical, mental and psychic perfection or *siddhi*.

Why is knowledge of anatomy and physiology useful for practitioners of pranayama?

Swami Niranjanananda: The best way to understand pranayama is to know human anatomy and physiology. Only then can a basic understanding of how pranayama works be gained.

After all, what is pranayama? Is it just the process of inhalation as described by Sage Patanjali? Is it just the process of exhalation, as described by Sage Patanjali? Is it just the process of retention as described by Sage Patanjali? The *Yoga Sutras* only say three things about pranayama – inhalation, exhalation and breath retention is pranayama. He doesn't say how to breathe, where to breathe, how long to breathe, what kind of pranayamas there are, other types of pranayamas that exist. He has spoken specifically on a general idea and on one specific pranayama in the *Yoga Sutras*. He has not covered the whole subject of pranayama, which is found in more detail in hatha yoga.

Hatha yoga describes the different practices of pranayama, like nadi shodhana, ujjayi, bhramari, kapalbhati, shanmukhi, plavini, bhastrika, sheetali, sheetkari – there are many practices of pranayama. People think that pranayama is just breathing in and breathing out and awakening the prana shakti. No, it is not like that, because each practice of pranayama fulfils a specific purpose for the development and awakening of the energy centres in the body, and every pranayama in the beginning, is associated with breath.

Through the regulation of the breath, one is asked to experience the activity and the motion of *pranayama*, of increasing the dimension of prana shakti – *prana*, the vital energy, plus *ayama*, to expand, to increase the dimension. The literal meaning of the word pranayama is increase of the dimension or area of vital energy. Respiration is a method by which one can begin to experience this prana shakti. How?

Prana is in everything, and in its relation to everything it has different names. The various manifestations of prana shakti have different waves, which are identified as bioplasmic, or electromagnetic waves that travel in the human body and are experienced in the body as an electrical current. There are different names for prana shakti according to the different manifestations in the environment, and within the body, in the different chakras. Prana is just the collective name of the energy in the universe and within us. When one begins to work with specific areas of respiration to induce a certain charge in the activity of the prana shakti, the different flows of prana are experienced.

When the breath is used, one needs to understand the anatomy and physiology of the lungs. The lungs are divided in three parts – the upper lobe, the middle lobe, and the lower lobe. In the middle and the lower lobes, there are alveoli, the air sacs of the lungs which allow for rapid gaseous exchange.

These lungs are separated from the digestive region by the diaphragm. The diaphragm is in an arched posture most of the time, so when one draws breath into the lower part of the lungs, allowing the breath to flow in the lower lobes, the diaphragm expands downwards, stimulating the digestive system by an increase in internal pressure. In pranayama, with the movement of breath in the different regions of the body, positive and negative pressures are created, activating a particular organ, or slowing down a particular function. Hence the breathing has been defined as thoracic breathing, or abdominal breathing, to indicate where the breath is moving in a particular pattern. In yogic breathing, there is an emphasis on breathing into the lower lobes of the lungs.

If pranayama is being practised to increase the vitality of the body, the oxygenation has to happen in a much simpler, smoother and easier way. Therefore, another thing that is emphasized in the practice of pranayama is absolute regulation of the breath – equal inhalation and equal exhalation. When one begins to control the breath, the breath is regulated and guided in a method which gives the experience of prana shakti.

When the positive and the negative pressures are created internally, the nerve plexuses are affected. This releases dormant or held back energy from within them, and a fresh burst of energy is felt. There are many scriptures, many literatures on pranayama, on swara yoga, on prana vidya, which describe the subject and the science of pranayama in detail, and also describe what prana is.

To study this subject properly it needs to be understood in relation to human anatomy and physiology. After all, one's body is a microcosmic experience. If the universe is macrocosmic, the body is a microcosmic universe. In this microcosmic universe, there are centres of energy, there are centres which correspond to the prithvi tattwa, the jala tattwa, and the other elements. In *prithvi tattwa*, the earth element, there is the energy of that element. One element is represented in each chakra, and each chakra is responsible for a specific manifestation of prana shakti. Each manifestation of prana shakti has a different colour, a different mode of perception. Therefore, this is not a subject that should be taken lightly. Rather, an in-depth study should be made by those who are keen to understand it.

Why should perspiration generated during pranayama be rubbed into the skin?

Swami Satyananda: When the body is unclean, impurities are excreted through the pores of the skin in the form of perspiration. When the body has been purified, only water, salt and hormones are excreted through the skin. When the body becomes hot due to pranayama, excess water may be lost. In the *Hatha Yoga Pradipika* (2:13) it is said:

Jalena shramajaatena gaatramardanamaacharet;
Dridhataa laghutaa chaiva tena gaatrasya jaayate.

Rub the body with the perspiration from the labour (of pranayama). The body derives firmness and steadiness from this, siddhi is attained.

There are seven dhatu known as *sapta dhatu*: blood, fat, flesh, bone, marrow, skin, semen/ova. To maintain these, certain hormones are produced, and when they cannot be stored they are expelled from the system. If there is perspiration due to pranayama, hormones are released unnecessarily. Therefore, the perspiration should be rubbed back into the skin so that they are reabsorbed through the pores. This helps to rebalance the system and tone the nerves and muscles.

PLACE OF PRACTICE

What environment is most suitable for a dedicated prana-yama sadhana?

Swami Sivananda: Select a solitary, beautiful and pleasant spot where there are no disturbances; on the bank of a river, lake or sea or the top or foot of a hill where there is a nice spring and grove of trees, or in a secluded part of a pleasant and beautiful garden. It is essential that the place is free from chills and strong draughts, mosquitoes, bugs, ants and all other flies or crawling insects.

Any such place where the unconcentrated mind easily becomes concentrated due to the presence of exceptionally good spiritual vibrations is ideal. Milk and articles of food should also be easily procurable. In India, the banks of the Ganges, the Jamuna and the Kaveri are extremely favourable for the practice of pranayama. Rishikesh, Vrindavan, Benares, Uttarkashi and Ayodhya are all very nice places for the purpose.

Those who practise in their own houses can convert a room into a forest. The room in which pranayama is practised should be dry and airy, it must not be damp or ill-ventilated. Never allow anyone to enter the room, not even one's dearest and nearest friends and relatives. Keep it under lock and key. Keep it sacred. If it is not possible to have a special room for contemplative purposes and for practising pranayama, have a place in the corner of a quiet room set apart for this purpose. Have it screened. Place the photo of your guru, favourite saint or deity in the room in front of the practice area.

In the selected place, seated in your favourite asana with the mind firmly fixed on truth, perform pranayama daily. Then the *chitta* or the mind-stuff gets absorbed in the sushumna. The prana becomes steady; it does not fluctuate. In the *Yoga Chudamani Upanishad* (v.106) it is written:

Baddhapadmaasano yogee namaskritya gurum shivam;
Naasaagra drishtirikaakee praanaayaamam samabhyaset.

Retiring to a solitary place, the yogi should sit in baddha padmasana, with the gaze fixed on the nosetip. Paying homage to the guru, who is Shiva, he should practise pranayama properly.

What type of place is best for practising pranayama?

Swami Niranjanananda: Pranayama should be practised in a clean environment to minimize the effects of pollution. One may practise in the open air or in a well-ventilated, clean and pleasant room. One should never perform pranayama in a foul-smelling, smoky or dusty room. Ideally, the place of practice should be somewhat isolated, away from people, noise and interruptions. Avoid practising in the sun or wind. The soft rays of the early morning sun are beneficial, but when they become stronger, they are harmful and the body will become overheated. Practising in a draught or wind may cause chills and upset the body temperature.

Pranayama should be practised every day at the same time and in the same place. This builds up positive, spiritual vibrations in the place, and the regularity creates inner strength and willpower.

What type of place is traditionally required for intensive pranayama sadhana?

Swami Niranjanananda: Sage Gheranda describes the environment for pranayama in detail in *Gheranda Samhita* (5:3–7):

Dooradeshe tathaa'ranye raajadhaanyaam janaantike;
Yogaarambham na kurveeta kritashchetsiddhihaa bhavet.

Avishvaasam dooradeshe aranye rakshivarjitam;
Lokaaranye prakaashashcha tasmaattreenivivarjayet.

Sudeshe dhaarmike raajye subhikshe nirupadrave;
Kritvaa tatraikam kuteeram praacheeraih pariveshtitam.

Vaapee koopatadaagam cha praacheera madhyavarti cha;
Naatyuchcham naatinimnam cha kuteeram keetavarjitam.

Samyaggomayaliptam cha kuteeram tatra nirmitam;
Evam sthaaneshu gupteshu praanaayaamam samabhyaset.

Yogic practices should not be done in a far-off place, in a forest, in a capital city or in a crowd, otherwise there

98

will be loss of siddhi, lack of success. Far-off places are forbidden because no one can be believed in a distant country, a forest is an insecure place, and in a capital city there is excessive population. Therefore, all three places are prohibited for pranayama. It should be done in a beautiful spiritual region, where food is readily available and the country is free from internal or external disturbances. Making a hut there, construct a boundary around it. There should be a well or a water source. The ground on which that hut is constructed should be neither too high nor too low, plastered with cow dung, free from insects and in a secluded place. Pranayama should be practised there. (3–7)

Sage Gheranda says that pranayama should not be practised in a distant country, forest or in a capital city which has undue light and noise due to the large population. For the practice of pranayama both an absolutely secluded place and an overcrowded place are prohibited. Sage Gheranda says that a new practitioner must observe these rules strictly.

If doing the practices in distant forests, a practitioner will not have the support of other people but if practising in an overcrowded city, everyone will watch. Therefore, the choice of either place is wrong. The point to be borne in mind is that in ancient times it was thought that an ordinary person should not obtain this yogic knowledge. Therefore Sage Gheranda, according to his thinking, has instructed that a practitioner should construct a hut in a peaceful spiritual place, where food products are easily available and there are no conflicts.

He says there should be a boundary wall around the hut and that within that boundary wall there should be a well or a small pond for the water supply. This is the main requirement of a practitioner. Wherever one lives, one should have enough water. Swami Satyananda used to say, "The place does not make any difference. Whether there is a house or trees does not matter, but there should be sufficient water, because water quenches the thirst and pure air flows in the water complex. When air is in contact with water, it causes the humidity and temperature to be favourable."

Sage Gheranda says the ground on which the hut is constructed should be neither too high nor too low and there should be no animals there. Once again he is educating aspirants on purity. The place should be plastered with cow dung, which is a pure substance that helps keep away insects and is easily kept clean, and it should be away from noise and disturbances.

Sage Gheranda gave these instructions according to the needs of that era and the feelings of those people. In the present era, when yoga has become quite common, when the population is increasing, and even pilgrimage places are becoming polluted, the place of practice should be selected with much consideration.

TIMING

Are the season and time of day important for pranayama sadhana?

Swami Sivananda: The practice of pranayama should be commenced in spring or autumn, because in these seasons success is attained without any difficulty or trouble. In the summer do not practise pranayama in the afternoon or evening. The cool morning hours are suitable for practice.

Suryabheda and ujjayi pranayamas produce heat. Sheetkari and sheetali are cooling. Bhastrika preserves normal temperature. Suryabheda destroys excess wind; ujjayi, phlegm; sheetkari and sheetali, bile; and bhastrika destroys all three. Suryabheda and ujjayi must be practised during winter. Sheetkari and sheetali must be practised in summer. Bhastrika can be practised in all seasons. Those persons whose bodies are hot even in winter can practise sheetkari and sheetali during the winter.

Pranayama should not be practised just after taking meals or when one is very hungry. A pranayama practitioner should take his food when pingala is working (when the breath flows through the right nostril), because pingala is heating and digests the food quickly.

In the beginning, have two sittings, morning and evening. As the practices advance, have four: morning, midday, evening and midnight.

Also, whenever one feels uneasy, depressed or dejected, practise pranayama. This will immediately bring a new vigour, energy and strength. The feelings will be elevated, renovated and filled with joy. Before writing something – an essay, an article or a thesis – do pranayama first. It will bring out beautiful ideas and the work will be an inspiring, powerful and original production.

How is pranayama practice affected by the seasons?

Swami Niranjanananda: There are no restrictions for those who are regular yoga practitioners, but when starting the practices, commence during spring or autumn, when the weather is fresh and it is neither too hot nor too cold.

In *Gheranda Samhita* (5:8–9 and 5:15) Sage Gheranda gives detailed instructions regarding the season during which pranayama practices should be undertaken. These are summarized in verses (8–9):

Hemante shishire greeshme varshaayaam cha ritau tathaa;
Yogaarambham na kurveeta krite yogo hi rogadah.

Vasante sharadi proktam yogaarambham samaacharet;
Tadaa yogee bhavetsiddho rogaanmukto bhaveddhruvam.

Yogic practices should not be commenced during winter, extreme cold, summer or the rainy season. If yogic practices are undertaken during these seasons, it leads to the spread of diseases. (8)

It is correct to start the practices during spring and autumn. When yogic practices are undertaken during these seasons, one certainly attains success and becomes free from diseases. (9)

Incidentally, these recommendations apply not only to practising pranayama, but also for the other yogic practices. The rules regarding the seasons are clear. It is said that yogic practices should not be commenced during summer, monsoon and winter. That is, when the temperature is extremely cold or extremely hot, or during the rains when the weather fluctuates from cold to hot.

Sage Gheranda warns that if the practices are begun during these times diseases will manifest. Diseases do manifest during this period if yogic practices are undertaken, particularly in the case of pranayama. If the weather is disregarded when commencing the practices, then due to the heat that is generated, boils, fever, the common cold, etc., tend to develop.

Yoga practices should be commenced during spring and autumn, as then the yogi attains perfection and diseases are removed. It is essential for the body to be able to adjust to, and be in harmony with, the changes that take place internally as a result of yogic practices, otherwise problems will arise. If yogic practices are begun when the weather is right, the body, environment and atmosphere are also favourable, one can bear with the changes taking place in the body and mind. Tolerance also increases, and so this change has a positive effect. If there is no tolerance, there will be a negative effect.

This point is made strongly by Sage Gheranda, who repeats the general advice in *Gheranda Samhita* (5:15):

Vasante vaapi sharadi yogaarambham samaacharet;
Tadaa yogo bhavetsiddho vinaa'yaasena kathyate.

It has been said that one attains success by commencing yogic practices during spring and autumn.

Sage Gheranda considers spring, *vasanta* and autumn, *sharada*, when it is moderately cold, to be the best seasons for commencing pranayama because only during these seasons can it be practised without obstacles. The number of pranayamas should also be reduced or increased according to the weather.

How does pranayama practice need to be adjusted according to the seasons?

Swami Niranjanananda: Normally in yoga, pranayama is divided into three parts. First, there are those pranayamas which generate heat and activity in the body and enhance the activity of the sympathetic nervous system. In the second group are those pranayamas which provide coolness, calmness and a state of relaxation to the body, and enhance the activity of the parasympathetic nervous system. The third group comprises those pranayamas which balance the activities of both the sympathetic and parasympathetic nervous systems. The instructions state that the third group of pranayamas can be practised during any month, because they are helpful in balancing the body's activity and temperature.

Those practices which enhance heat in the body are mostly undertaken during cold weather and those practices which cool the body are performed during hot weather. That is why hatha yoga says that pranayamas should be practised according to the seasons.

For regular practitioners season need not be a barrier or obstacle to the practices. When one becomes established in the advanced practices, their effects are by no means unnatural for the sadhaka. Pranayama remains beneficial as it has become part of the daily routine. Therefore, the advice on seasonal adjustments is not meant for experienced practitioners.

Do the scriptures recommend certain times of day for the practice of pranayama?

Swami Satyananda: In *Hatha Yoga Pradipika* (2:11) it is said:

Praatarmadhyadine saayamardharaatre cha kumbhakaan;
Shanairasheetiparyantam chaturvaaram samabhyaset.

Retention should be practised perfectly four times a day: early morning, midday, evening and midnight, so that retention is gradually held up to eighty (counts in one sitting).

Those who are completely dedicated to a life of hatha sadhana should practise pranayama at the four specified times, but due to the nature of modern social commitments and the way of life, few would find this possible. For the average person it is sufficient to practise once a day. It is best to rise early in the morning, take a bath, do neti and kunjal if necessary, then practise asanas and pranayama. If there is the opportunity to do sadhana in the evening, do it before eating.

The specified times for practice are important in relation to body rhythms and solar and lunar activities. At these times there is a change over of body and external energy rhythms, and sushumna nadi is more likely to become active.

Early morning means an hour and a half before sunrise. It is called *brahmamuhurta*, 'the period of Brahma'. At this time the subconscious mind is active and if one is sleeping there are likely to be dreams. It is a time when unconscious experiences are more likely to manifest.

Evening, around the time of sunset, is called sandhya. *Sandhya* is the meeting of day and night. It represents the time when ida and pingala merge with sushumna in ajna chakra. The external influences of the sun setting, or the evening commencing, affect body rhythms and functions, making it conducive to the merging of the pranas in sushumna.

Similarly, at midnight and midday there is a changeover in the external and internal energies. All becomes tranquil. Midnight in particular is the time for sadhakas to awaken shakti. It is called the 'witching hour' because the 'ghosts' in the mind become active. Brain functions operate differently at night and different chemical hormones are released.

At these specified times there is a change in the levels of energy in ida and pingala. During each cycle of ida and pingala there are high and low phases when energy reaches either a peak or a low. In between each cycle there is a period when the energy is stable, and this is the most appropriate time for sadhana and breath retention. The times recommended for the practice of retention have been chosen on account of the biological and pranic activities that are taking place then.

For most people, it is not advisable to practise pranayama at midnight unless specified by the guru. If one practises then, it will disturb the normal pattern of living and those living in the same dwelling will consider the practitioner absurd. Also, because the unconscious mind becomes active at this time, if negative impressions come to the surface there might be frightening experiences which are difficult to cope with.

If one practises pranayama in the morning or evening and lives a simple life, the pure thoughts will exorcize these 'ghosts' so that positive experiences unfold. Until the mind and body are purified, go slowly with practices according to the guru's instructions. Do not be over enthusiastic.

Pranayama should be done in correct proportion to other practices and one's routine daily activities. Other forms of yoga should be integrated into the sadhana so that there is a balanced development of the personality. A person who goes headlong into sadhana cannot maintain the schedule for many years. Sadhana should be gradually increased according to time available and one's mental, physical, and psychic capacity.

What time of day is best for pranayama?
Swami Niranjanananda: The yogic texts advise four periods for the practice of pranayama: sunrise, noon, sunset and midnight, but this is for advanced practitioners only. Early morning is the best time to practise pranayama. At the time of *brahmamuhurta*, between 4 and 6 am, the vibrations of the atmosphere are in their purest state. The body is fresh and the mind has few impressions compared to its state at

105

the end of the day. Most pranayamas should not be done in the heat of the day, unless a special sadhana is given by the guru.

Another reason for doing practices in the morning is the quality of the atmosphere early in the day. Electrically-charged particles in the atmosphere, called negative ions, are fewer during the daytime due to the heat. Their reduced number means that at the time of pranayama the body cannot experience energy and agility, and instead stress and distress may be experienced. There is freshness in the early morning environment, indicating a high number of negatively charged ions in the air. By doing pranayama at that time, those ions full of electrical energy enter the body and provide energy and vitality.

Pranayama should not be practised after meals. One must wait for three hours after a meal before practising. An empty stomach ensures that the prana vayus are not concentrated in the digestive process and can be used to initiate more subtle activities. At the same time, pranayama should not be practised when one is hungry.

In the evening if the pranas are active in our system, they are not in a state of harmony. So it is better to do pranayama in the morning to feel revitalized. Of course it is advisable to do it in the evening also – do it at both times, but one should not continue pranayama practice when fatigued. There must always be joy and exhilaration during and after the practice. One should come out of the practice fully invigorated and refreshed.

SEQUENCE OF PRACTICE

How long does it take to learn pranayama?
Swami Satyananda: Prana opens the secret doors of the mind and experience, and pranayama explodes the hidden phases of energy in the human mind and body. But for this, it must be properly practised. The body and various organs have to be brought under perfect control.

Prana is a wild elephant. If it has not been tamed, it can be disastrous. Therefore, before the practice of pranayama, the hatha yoga *shatkarmas*, the six processes of purification, must be practised. Before pranayama, the asanas should be perfected, and before the higher practices of pranayama, the diet must be reduced to a minimum. An aspirant of pranayama does not live to eat, but eats to live.

Pranayama must be practised for a sustained period until the whole brain and all the elements of the body are purified. One must not practice for one or two months only and then say, "Now I have learned pranayama". That's not enough. It's not just the learning of hatha yoga or the learning of pranayama, but the assimilation of the entire practice, the whole system, which is required.

Why does hatha yoga recommend practising shatkarmas before pranayama?

Swami Satyananda: Excess mucus is the major obstacle which prevents pranayama practice. If the body is clogged with old mucus, bile and wind, the energy generated through pranayama practice will be used for rectifying these disorders. For nasal congestion, neti and kunjal are sufficient, but for respiratory congestion such as asthma or bronchitis, laghoo shankhaprakshalana is also necessary. First the practitioner must rid himself of excess mucus and bile and eliminate the toxins from his system. Proper assimilation and excretion need to be established. Pranayama is more effective in a healthy body. In *Hatha Yoga Pradipika* (2:36) it is said:

Shatkarmanirgatasthaulyakaphadoshamalaadikah;
Praanaayaamam tatah kuryaadanaayaasena siddhyati.

By the six karmas (shatkarma) one is freed from excesses of the doshas. Then pranayama is practised and success is achieved without strain.

By practising pranayama correctly the mind is automatically conquered. However, the effects of pranayama are not so simple to manage. It creates extra heat in the body, it awakens some of the dormant centres in the brain, it can alter the production of sperm and testosterone. It lowers the respiratory rate and changes the brainwave patterns. When these changes take place the aspirant may not be able to handle it. For this reason also, hatha yoga says first purify the body by the practice of shatkarmas.

Shatkarma provides a quick method of rebalancing mucus, bile and wind. If the body is cleansed through shatkarma first, pranayama will maintain the state of cleanliness. However, if the body is already healthy, nadis clean and the whole system is functioning in harmony, then pranayama can be practised without any need for shatkarma. If there is a slight imbalance, pranayama alone will be sufficient to rectify any problems.

What is the role of asanas and shatkarmas when preparing for pranayama practice?
Swami Niranjanananda: In order to qualify for pranayama one must first master yoga asanas. In order to reap the full benefit of asanas, one must undergo the process of shatkarmas. The physical body is a combination and permutation of the five elements: earth, water, fire, air and ether. Shatkarmas purify these elements, so that they do not interfere with the activities of prana. The effect of asanas and pranayamas increases substantially when the body is relieved of toxins. The body becomes sensitive and responds to the changes that an asana or pranayama demands from it.

The inner body of a pranayama practitioner needs to be pure. Adverse effects may be experienced if one practises pranayama without removing the energy blocks and toxins accumulated on account of an irregular lifestyle. For example, fermentation of mucus will immediately interfere with pranic activities. The practice of shatkarmas gives a good flushing to the mouth, nose, stomach, intestines, and indeed the whole alimentary canal.

When shatkarmas are followed by asanas, the pranas are able to penetrate each and every nerve, cell and pore of the body. The practitioner will reap enormous benefits by following a routine of shatkarmas, asanas and pranayamas, even if he has completely neglected the body for years. However, if one has led a simple and balanced lifestyle, and maintained purity of the body, then one can start directly with pranayama.

Why is pranayama practised after asanas and before meditation?

Swami Niranjanananda: By performing pranayama after asana practice, the physiological and pranic systems are relaxed and balanced. After doing asanas, the practitioner may rest for five minutes and then begin pranayama. There are some practitioners to whom the guru suggests the practice of pranayama before asanas, but this only happens in a few cases and is done under the guidance of the guru. The common sequence is asana first, pranayama second, and the other practices of relaxation and meditation following that. The mind becomes one-pointed and the body feels lighter after pranayama. This makes meditation more enjoyable. In *Hatharatnavali* (3:78) it is written:

> *Athaasane dridhe yogee vashee hitamitaashanah;*
> *Guroopadishtamaargena praanaayaamaansamabhyaset.*

After becoming well-versed in asanas, the yogi with his senses under control and eating moderate agreeable food, should practise pranayama as advised by the guru.

POSTURE

What is the ideal sitting posture for the practice of pranayama?

Swami Sivananda: Correct posture is an indispensable requisite for the successful practice of pranayama. Asana means an easy comfortable posture. The best pose is the one which continues to be comfortable for the greatest length of time. Chest, neck and head must be in one vertical line, so that the spinal cord which lies within the spinal column is quite free. The body should not bend either forwards or backwards or to the right or left side. In *Hatharatnavali* (3:84) it says:

Siddhe vaa baddhapadme vaa svastikevaabhavaasane;
Rijukaayah samaaseenah praanaayaamaansamabhyaset.

Pranayama should be practised in siddhasana, baddha padmasana or swastikasana, sitting on level ground with the body erect.

Why are specific types of mat and posture recommended for pranayama?

Swami Niranjanananda: Natural fibres such as cotton or wool are best to sit on for the practice of pranayama. It is not advisable to sit on or wear materials made of synthetic fibres, as they repel negative ions and attract positive ions. Positive ions are not conducive to pranayama or to good health because they act as a shield, obstructing the flow of negative ions into the body. Traditionally, a mat of kusha, sacred grass, was used. In *Shiva Samhita* (3:20) it is written:

Sushobhane mathe yogee padmaasanasamanvitah;
Aasanopari samvishya pavanaabhyaasamaacharet.

Let the yogi go to a beautiful and pleasant place of retirement or a cell, assume the posture padmasana, and sitting on a seat made of kusha grass, begin to practise the regulation of the breath.

The ability to sit comfortably in a meditation asana is a prerequisite for the successful practice of pranayama. The correct posture enables efficient breathing as well as stability of the body. Both concentration and technique are hampered by poor posture. One should not allow the body to become crooked or to collapse. By regular practice, mastery over the pose will come by itself.

The best postures for the practice of pranayama are padmasana, siddhasana, siddha yoni asana and swastikasana. When one advances in the practice, prana moves through the body at a terrific speed. This movement must be supported by total immobility of the body, which these postures maintain. As the body produces more energy, it effectively turns into an electrical pole. The left side carries cool energy and the right warm energy, representing the negative and positive poles. The additional energy produced by the practice can escape through the earth connection. Therefore, a closed circuit must be created to ensure that the energy remains within the body. This circuit is made by these four meditation postures, and strengthened by the application of mudras and bandhas. This may not apply to a beginner, but if one wants to advance in pranayama, then expertise in the meditation asanas is imperative. In the beginning however, one may sit in *sukhasana*, the easy pose, especially if one is overweight.

What simple pranayama can be practised in shavasana?

Swami Sivananda: Those who are very weak can practise pranayama in the pose of shavasana while lying on the ground or on a bed. The breath should be drawn in slowly, without making any noise, through both nostrils, and retained for as long as is comfortable, before exhaling very slowly through both nostrils. Repeat the process twelve times in the morning and twelve times in the evening. Chant *Om* mentally during the practice. This is a combined exercise of asana, pranayama, meditation and rest. It gives rest not only to the body but also to the mind. It gives relief, comfort and ease. This is suitable for aged people.

How can pranayama be practiced while walking?

Swami Sivananda: Walk with head up, shoulders back and the chest expanded. Inhale slowly through both nostrils counting *Om* mentally three times, one count for each step. Then retain the breath for twelve counts of *Om*. Then exhale slowly through both nostrils for six counts of *Om*. If it is difficult to count *Om* with each step, count *Om* without any concern for the steps.

Kapalabhati can also be done during walking. Those who are very busy can practise the above pranayama during their morning and evening walks. It is like killing two birds with one stone. It is most pleasant to practise pranayama while walking in an open place, when a delightful gentle breeze is blowing. An invigorating effect occurs quickly and to a considerable degree. Practise, feel and realize the marked, beneficial influence of this kind of pranayama. Those who walk briskly, repeating *Om* mentally or verbally, are practising natural pranayama without any effort.

DIET

What is the best diet for pranayama practitioners?

Swami Sivananda: Foods detrimental to the practice of yoga should be abandoned. Give up salt, mustard, sour, hot, pungent and bitter things. The diet should be light and moderate, with no emaciation of the body by fasts. In the early stages, milk and ghee are advised; foods made from wheat, green pulse and red rice are said to favour progress.

What dietary advice does hatha yoga give for pranayama practitioners?

Swami Niranjanananda: The sages have thoughtfully pre-scribed some dietary rules from ancient times. In *Gheranda Samhita* Sage Gheranda says that pranayama practitioners should eat a moderate, balanced diet, otherwise the full benefit of the practices will not be derived. Also, eating unsuitable or unseasonable food leads to the possibility of physical ailments. Wherever discussion about diet or food takes place, these rules about which vegetables or fruits should be taken during monsoon or winter are considered. Thus, for each season a different type of food is recommended. These rules are particularly observed in

112

villages. In the modern era, with refrigeration, people have begun keeping and preserving out of season vegetables and fruits, but according to yoga, consuming unseasonable food has detrimental effects on the body. This is specified in *Gheranda Samhita* (5:16):

Mitaahaaram vinaa yastu yogaarambham tu kaarayet;
Naanaarogo bhavettasyakinchidyogo na sidhyati.

A practitioner who undertakes yoga without moderating the diet suffers from many diseases and does not make progress in yoga.

Furthermore, Sage Gheranda says that a sadhaka should eat less and should consume a balanced diet, specifying the following foods. Rotis or chapatis made by mixing rice, wheat, barley, grams and urad dal are considered best for yogis. Vegetables and fruits like jackfruit, parval, bitter gourd (karela), eggplant (brinjal), cucumber, figs, unripe bananas (plantain), etc., can also be eaten. Seasonal green vegetables are useful. In fact, a wide range of food is beneficial for pranayama, because when pranayama is practised, heat is generated in the body, which starts to dissolve any excess fat. That is why pranayama practitioners take ghee (clarified butter), so that the body fat which is reduced during pranayama is replenished.

Sage Gheranda has also prescribed rules regarding the quantity of food to be taken. It is said that not too much food should be eaten. The rule for food intake is that half the stomach should be filled with food, one quarter with water, and the remaining one quarter should be left empty for the circulation of air. Eating until the stomach is full is prohibited. Thus, physical health is maintained by consuming food which causes no discomfort or stomach problems. These rules are given in *Gheranda Samhita* (5:21–22):

Shuddham sumadhuram snigdhamudaraardhavivarjitam;
Bhujyate surasampreetyaa mitaahaaramimam viduh.

Annena poorayedardham toyena tu triteeyakam;
Udarasya tureeyaamsham samrakshedvaayuchaarane.

The stomach should be half-filled with pleasing, pure, sweet, cooling, oily or lubricating materials until satisfied, and half of the stomach should be left empty. Learned people have termed it mitahara, meaning balance, control or moderation in eating. (21)

Half of the stomach should be filled with food, a quarter with water and the fourth quarter left empty for the circulation of air. (22)

What foods are prohibited during pranayama practice?

Swami Niranjanananda: In *Gheranda Samhita* (5:23–31) Sage Gheranda talks about food products and certain behaviours that are forbidden for serious pranayama practitioners:

Katvamlam lavanam tiktam bhrishtam cha dadhitakrakam;
Shaakotkatam tathaa madyam taalam cha panasam tathaa.

Kulattham masuram paandum kooshmaandam shaakadandakam;
Tumbeekolakapittham cha kantabilvam palaashakam.

Kadambam jambeeram bimbam lakucham lashunam visham;
Kaamarangam piyaalam cha hingushaalmalikemukam.

Yogaarambhe varjayechcha pathistreevahnisevanam.
Navaneetam ghritam ksheeram sharkaraadyaikshavam gudam;

Pakvarambhaam naarikelam daadimbamashivaasavam;
Draakshaam tu lavaleem dhaatreem rasamamlavivarjitam.

When commencing yogic practice one should avoid bitter, sour or acidic, salty and astringent foods, fried food, curd, buttermilk, heavy vegetables, wine, palm nuts and overripe jackfruit. Consuming foods such as horse gram and lentils, pandu fruit, pumpkin and vegetable stems, gourds, berries, limes, garlic, asafoetida, etc., are prohibited. (23–25)

114

A beginner should avoid excess travelling, the company of women or warming himself by the fire. Fresh butter, clarified butter, milk, jaggery, sugar, amalaki, pomegranate, grapes, ripe bananas, etc., should also not be used. (26–27)

It is not known on what pretext, but he mentions here that a male practitioner on the yogic path should avoid the company of women or warming himself by the fire. Maybe he has prescribed this as an external discipline in order to maintain internal control, because initially the sexual urge increases as heat is generated in the body by pranayama practice. When a person practises in a secluded place or under the direction of a guru, he can maintain inner control, but if he does not stay in an isolated place and the guru is also not close by, it is possible to lose control in the heat of the moment. Maybe that is why Sage Gheranda has repeated these rules for observing physical control and celibacy.

He goes on to state that it is not beneficial for yogis to eat either cold or very hot foods, which cause extreme changes in body temperature. Here it can be mentioned for today's students that chilled water should not be drunk immediately after pranayama or dynamic exercise, or on coming in from the sun. Water should be normal temperature, not chilled. It should be left for at least five to ten minutes if it has been chilled. This is recommended in order to maintain normal body temperature.

Elaajaatilavangam cha paurusham jambujaambalam;
Hareetakeem cha kharjooram yogee bhakshanamaacharet.

Laghupaakam priyam snigdham tathaa dhaatupraposhanam;
Mano'bhilashitam yogyam yogee bhojanamaacharet;
Kathinam duritam pootimushnam paryushitam tathaa;
Atisheetam chaatichoshnam bhakshyam yogee vivarjayet.

Praatahsnaanopavaasaadi kaayakleshavidhim tathaa;
Ekaahaaram niraahaaram yaamaante cha na kaarayet.

Evam vidhi vidhaanena praanaayaamam samaacharet;
Aarambhe prathame kuryaatksheeraajyam nityabhojanam;
Madhyaahne chaiva saayaahne bhojanadvayamaacharet.

Cardamom, cloves, nutmeg, stimulants, haritaki and dates can be taken. (28)

Only foods which are easily digestible, agreeable, lubricating, strengthening and acceptable to the mind should be eaten. Hard, polluted, stale, heating, extremely cold and extremely hot foods should be avoided. (29)

Early morning bathing and fasting, which cause discomfort to the body, should be discarded. Having only one meal a day, not eating at all or eating between meals should be discontinued. (30)

Prior to commencing pranayama practice, one should have milk and ghee daily and eat two meals a day, one at noon and one in the evening. (31)

Sage Gheranda also says that a pranayama practitioner should not eat sour, acidic or overly salted foods, or condiments and fried foods in excess. Beginners should not consume curd or sour vegetables, onions, cauliflower, etc. The food products mentioned are native to India, but one must use common sense and avoid foods which tend to increased *pitta* (acidity) or produce gas.

In describing such rules Sage Gheranda says that *vata*, gas, *pitta*, heat, and *kapha*, mucus, related to the digestive system should be kept under control and not aggravated. Milk produces kapha, so here Sage Gheranda is overturning the normal idea that yogis should drink a lot of milk. He also lists ginger, sugar and dried fruits, the specific reason being that there should be no excessive desire for taste sensations.

Cardamom, cloves, haritaki, etc., can be used as they help in the digestion of food. He has permitted the use of pure ghee, but not the use of butter. Ghee is made by heating

116

butter and skimming off the white foam so that only pure ghee remains. The foam in butter hides the sour taste which increases acidity or pitta in the body.

To summarize, food should be easily digestible, light and energy producing. The stomach should not feel heavy or the body lethargic after eating.

Sage Gheranda says that one should not bathe immediately before or after pranayama practice. If the body temperature drops and pranayama is practised immediately afterwards, it will have an adverse effect. The normal rule is to practise asanas after bathing in order to normalize the body temperature before pranayama practice. If this routine is followed, bathing prior to pranayama practice is valid and justified.

Sage Gheranda says that fasting for more than twenty-four hours should not be observed as pranayama creates heat in the body and the body needs to be strong to maintain the practice. However, he also says that fasting for one meal a day can be done. This will at least enable the body to maintain some energy. Eating snacks between meals is not beneficial.

Finally, Sage Gheranda says that milk can be taken. First he has forbidden the drinking of milk and then he says that milk can be taken along with food. From this it can be inferred that milk should probably not be taken on an empty stomach. Milk is digested when taken with food and does not remain inside the stomach. If it is taken at night time before sleeping, it remains in the stomach and the nutritional elements of the milk are not digested properly due to dominance of the parasympathetic nervous system.

In summary, a yogi should observe these main rules. First of all pranayama should be practised. Then milk and ghee should be taken with food. Food should be taken regularly but only twice, once in the morning and once in the evening.

Why is drinking milk recommended during pranayama sadhana?

Swami Satyananda: When a sadhaka starts to practise pranayama the body metabolism undergoes a change. The heart rate and blood pressure are activated and all body processes are energized. Digestive secretions and excretory processes are stimulated. To help maintain balance until the body adjusts, it is advised to take milk because it has a neutralizing effect on the body and helps lubricate the system. Milk products help increase the fats which are important for insulating the body when the prana is increased. Otherwise, if fats are quickly used one may 'blow a fuse' in the energy system. If the fats are burnt up before they are distributed, lymphatic mechanisms are increased. The lymphatic system releases fats into the body from the digestive tract. Pranayama directly affects this mechanism. In *Hatha Yoga Pradipika* (2:14) it is said:

> *Abhyaasakaale prathame shastam ksheeraajyabhojanam;*
> *Tato'bhyaase dridheebhoote na taadrinniyamagrahah.*

> In the beginning stages of practice, food consisting of milk and ghee is recommended. Upon being established in the practice such restrictions are not necessary.

There is another important factor; milk contains animal proteins which have a direct effect on the body and mind. Pranayama can awaken an altered state of consciousness, but the animal proteins help maintain normal conscious functioning. If psychic experiences occur too rapidly, before the mind is ready, there will be difficulties coping. Once the whole system is adjusted, it is not necessary to take milk.

When should the pranayama practitioner eat?

Swami Satyananda: When practising pranayama the stomach must be completely empty, and after the practice food should not be taken for at least half an hour. Light, easily digestible and nourishing food facilitates pranayama practice.

What are the dietary recommendations when practising pranayama?

Swami Niranjanananda: The practitioner of pranayama should choose a balanced diet that is suitable to his constitution. There is no one diet that is right or wrong for everyone. As the saying goes, 'One man's food is another man's poison'.

Food can be classified into three basic groups: i) tamasic – which creates lethargy, dullness; ii) rajasic – which creates excitement, passion and disease, and iii) sattwic – which bestows balance, good health and longevity. Fresh and natural foods are sattwic; packaged and refined foods are tamasic and should be avoided.

A diet of grains, pulses, fresh fruit and vegetables, and a small amount of dairy products is most beneficial. For non-vegetarians, a small portion of meat, fish or eggs may be added. The diet must also be adjusted to avoid constipation. Overall, the principle of moderation should be followed.

The Ayurvedic principle in regard to diet is: fill half the stomach with food, one quarter with water and leave one quarter empty. Given the opportunity, most people overeat, when they could manage better on one balanced meal per day. Excessive eating satisfies the senses and the mind, but it places pressure on the diaphragm and lungs, and full-depth respiration becomes difficult.

PRECAUTIONS

Are there any dangers in practising pranayama?

Swami Sivananda: There is no danger in practising pranayamas if one is careful, and if common sense is used. People are unnecessarily alarmed. There is danger in everything if one is careless. The *Yoga Chudamani Upanishad* (v. 118) states:

Yathaa simho gajo vyaaghro bhavedvashyah shanaih shanaih;
Tathaiva sevito vaayuranyathaa hanti saadhakam.

119

Just as the lion, elephant and tiger are brought under control slowly and steadily, similarly the prana should be controlled, otherwise it becomes destructive to the practitioner.

What precautions should the pranayama practitioner be aware of?

Swami Niranjanananda: The lungs, heart and nerves are normally strong and gain added strength with regulated and sensible pranayama practice. However, if the practitioner overdoes it or performs unsuitable practices, the body may be weakened and the inner organs damaged. Pranayama also accentuates whatever is in the mind, whether positive or negative. So, by wrong or excessive practice, one's mental quirks and even nervous tics could become exaggerated. *Hatha Yoga Pradipika* (2:16) states:

Praanaayaamena yuktena sarvarogakshayo bhavet;
Ayuktaabhyaasayogena sarvarogasamudbhavah.

All diseases are eradicated by the proper practice of pranayama; all diseases can arise through improper practice.

When pranayama is improperly practised, problems may arise without any warning signals, so extra care is required. Every practice should be treated with respect and caution.

There should be no violent respirations, no extended kumbhaka beyond a comfortable measure, no forcing of the breath, body or mind. The practitioner should not attempt to perform an advanced pranayama which is beyond his present capabilities. In this way comfortable progress will be assured and one will be able to achieve full benefit from the wonderful science of pranayama.

Is pranayama suitable for everyone?

Swami Niranjanananda: Pranayama can be practised by all people, regardless of age and physical condition.

However, the practices should be learned individually from a master or qualified teacher and not selected at random. Every individual has a different physical and mental constitution, which a qualified teacher is able to assess. Specific pranayamas, rounds and ratios are prescribed according to these criteria. These subtleties cannot be gauged without the maturity of practice and understanding.

THE SADHAKA

What personal qualities facilitate success in the practice of pranayama?

Swami Sivananda: One who has a calm mind, who has subdued his senses, who has faith in the words of the guru and scriptures, who believes in God, who is moderate in eating, drinking and sleeping, and who has an eager longing for deliverance from the wheel of birth and death, is well qualified for the practice of pranayama or any other yoga practice. Celibacy is ideal but if this is not possible then copulation should be kept to a minimum. Such a person can easily have success in the practice. Pranayama should be practised with care, perseverance and faith.

Those who are addicted to sensual pleasures or who are arrogant, dishonest, untruthful, cunning and treacherous; those who disrespect sadhus, sannyasins and their gurus or spiritual preceptors, and take pleasure in vain controversies or are of a highly talkative nature; those who are disbelievers, who mix much with worldly-minded people, who are cruel, harsh and greedy and do much useless worldly activity, can never attain success in pranayama or any other yoga practice.

The seeker must approach a guru who knows the science of yoga and has mastery over it. Sit at his lotus feet and serve him. Clear any doubts through sensible and reasonable questions. Receive instructions and practise them with enthusiasm, zeal, attention, earnestness and faith, according to the methods taught by the teacher.

There must always be joy and exhilaration of spirit during and after the practice. One should come out of the practice fully invigorated and refreshed. Take care not to be bound by too many rules. In *Shiva Samhita* (3:31) it is written:

Praudhavahnih subhogee cha sukhisarvaangasundarah;
Sampoornahridayo yogee sarvotsaahabalaanvitah;
Jaayate yogino'vashyametatsarvam kalevare.

The following qualities are surely always found in the bodies of every yogi: strong appetite, good digestion, cheerfulness, handsome figure, great courage, mighty enthusiasm and full strength.

How do the gunas influence the practice of pranayama?
Swami Satyananda: There are three modes of nature and mind known as the gunas: they are tamas, rajas and sattwa. *Tamas* is inertia, *rajas* is dynamism and *sattwa* is steadiness. For example, a rock represents tamas, man represents rajas and divinity represents sattwa. The dull mind, or the mind in which there is no awareness, is tamasic or inert; the mind which oscillates between awareness and no awareness is rajasic or dynamic; and the steady, one-pointed mind is sattwic. In *Hatha Yoga Pradipika* (2:6) it is written:

Praanaayaamam tatah kuryaannityam saattvikayaa dhiyaa;
Yathaa sushumnaanaadeesthaa malaah shuddhim prayaanti cha.

Therefore, pranayama should be done daily with a sattwic state of mind so that the impurities are driven out of sushumna nadi and purification occurs.

During pranayama practice the mind should be steady and aware, and not moving from thought to thought. Then the whole system is receptive. When the mind is inert or tamasic, some of the nadis remain inert and closed, impurities collect and the energy cannot pass. However, this does not mean that if one is tamasic, pranayama cannot be practised. Whether one is tamasic or rajasic, pranayama should be practised to remove the blockages and to lift the practitioner out of the tamasic and rajasic states. When the mind is sattwic, the inner awareness grows quickly and prana accumulates.

When sushumna awakens, this represents sattwa, when pingala functions it represents rajas and when ida functions, tamas. Thus it is best to practise pranayama when sushumna is flowing. When the breath is flowing naturally through both nostrils it means sushumna is active. We do not always breathe through both nostrils, usually one nostril is open and the other is partially or fully closed. Science calls it 'alternate rhinitis'. In yoga it is known as *swara*.

What is a simple pranayama sadhana for daily use?
Swami Niranjanananda: In one day five capsules of yoga have to be taken, eaten and digested. The first capsule of yoga is called vitamin mantra, and it is taken early in the morning. The second capsule of yoga is called vitamin asana, and it is taken before breakfast. The third capsule is vitamin pranayama, and it is also taken before breakfast. There are two practices of pranayama which are important.

In order to relax the nerves and bring a balance between the functions of the left and right hemispheres of the brain, to increase the vitality and stamina in the body, and to harmonize the dissipated energies, the first practice should be *nadi shodhana pranayama*, alternate nostril breathing. The breath should be equal during inhalation and exhalation. The seconds can be counted to regulate the length and the depth of inhalation and exhalation. Seven seconds breathing in through the left nostril, seven seconds breathing out through the right nostril, then again breathe in through the right for seven seconds and breathe out through the left for seven seconds. This is one round of the practice. About five to seven rounds should be practised.

The second pranayama is *bhramari* pranayama – humming like a bumble bee. Close the ears, breathe in deeply, and breathe out with a low humming. Practise this pranayama five to seven times. Bhramari helps regulate the endocrine system which regulates the hormones in the body. It improves concentration and awareness and is a preparation for higher stages of meditation as it helps internalize the sensory perceptions. Additionally, bhramari is useful for hypertension caused by stress in life. Much research has been done, showing this to be the only technique which can effectively lower high blood pressure.

The majority of stress-related problems can be managed with these two pranayamas: nadi shodhana and bhramari. This pranayama is the third capsule of yoga, which is needed before having breakfast.

The fourth capsule is yoga nidra in the afternoon, and the fifth is meditation just before sleeping.

Why should children be taught pranayama?

Swami Satyananda: Practically everybody should do pranayama, which is why in India pranayama practices were traditionally taught at the age of seven. When one starts pranayama at an early age one goes slowly, gradually, like a clock. Then by the age of thirty, thirty-four, forty-five, fifty, fifty-five, one can go into higher and deeper practices of pranayama in which the breath is held, and all the bandhas are performed, and experiences come. One must take time.

Why is single-minded concentration necessary during pranayama?

Swami Satyananda: During the practice of pranayama the mind has a natural tendency to run away in the multitude of thoughts and emotions which arise. This happens particularly during the practice of bhastrika pranayama. Thoughts come rapidly and the awareness is easily swept away by their force. It is not sufficient to merely perform pranayama mechanically, while the awareness is dissipating and rambling in the quagmire of illusory thoughts and visions, there must be concentration on the present moment. Mind, body and prana must cooperate together so that the three start to work in unison. Therefore, there has to be a method for concentration throughout the practice. In *Hatha Yoga Pradipika* (3:127) it is said:

Maarutasya vidhim sarvam manoyuktam samabhyaset;
Itaratra na kartavyaa manovrittirmaneeshinaa.

All the pranayama methods are to be done with a concentrated mind. The wise man should not let his mind be involved in the modifications (vrittis).

Single-minded concentration is essential in all the practices, whether pranayama, asana or mudra. It is the essence of perfection in every form of yoga. In every situation, not only while practising pranayama, one must pay attention and become aware of the experiences, actions and thoughts in that moment. Development of awareness whilst awake leads to constant awareness in the deeper states of dhyana and samadhi.

What attitude should the practitioner have towards progress in pranayama?

Swami Niranjanananda: Patience and perseverance are necessary in spiritual life, and this is especially true for pranayama. The practitioner should not be frustrated if he cannot attain a certain ratio or number of rounds; it may take months or even years to perfect one pranayama alone. The regular practitioner is progressing all the time although the progress cannot be seen objectively, so there is a tendency to think that nothing is happening. However, one should be assured that the practice is developing on both the gross and subtle levels.

One of the most important disciplines for the practitioner of pranayama is regularity. This means developing a regular lifestyle as well as being consistent in the practice of pranayama itself. There will be no progress if one jumps from one practice to another every day. In the beginning one should ask the teacher to create a capsule of daily pranayamas, which should be improved to a high degree through regular practice.

Pranayama practices progress over a period of time. Beginners need to practise the preliminaries in order to go on to the more advanced levels. Regularity in practice is essential for increasing the physiological capability as well as adjusting the body and mind to the increased pranic force. This is slow and steady process, and the practitioner should never try to hurry.

What is the advice for those undertaking serious pranayama sadhana?

Swami Satyananda: As one advances in the practice of pranayama, precautions have to be taken. 'Advances' here means one begins practising for durations of longer than twenty minutes and with extended breath retentions of more than thirty seconds. Steps to establish good health must be taken before commencing serious pranayama sadhana.

One should make the body strong by regular practice of asanas and ensure that the body is purified. Pranayama itself will do this, but the shatkarmas, such as shankhaprakshalana and neti, are perfectly suited for removing gross impurities. The importance of physical purity is indicated in the scriptures. In the *Yoga Chudamani Upanishad* (v. 94) it is said:

> *Shuddhimeti yadaa sarva naadeechakram malaakulam;*
> *Tadaiva jaayate yogee praanasangrahanakshamah.*

> When all the nadis and chakras become free from their accumulation of impurities, then only the yogi becomes capable of controlling the breath.

Another important point, essential in fact, is that one must eat pure and vegetarian food. Failure to do this could easily lead to harm and disease. For those who are practising a lot of pranayama, the adoption of a simple, balanced and pure diet is vital. Also, serious pranayama should not be practised when one is ill.

It is advised that those who are practising a lot of pranayama should do so under the guidance of a competent teacher. Pranayama is a powerful technique if it is done correctly; but if a lot of pranayama is done incorrectly, it will cause harm.

The one who masters pranayama masters the mind. In *Hatha Yoga Pradipika* (4:29) it says, *Indriyaanaam mano naatho manonaathastu maarutah*, "Mind is the ruler of the senses, and prana is the ruler of the mind . . ."

Pranayama itself can lead to awareness of the depths of the mind and beyond, but please don't overdo the practice. First practise gently for a few years in order to slowly accustom the physical and pranic bodies to new functional conditions. This point should be clearly understood and remembered.

What is the difference between prayanama sadhana and general pranayama practice?

Swami Niranjanananda: The pranayama usually taught by yoga teachers is only preparatory. The main purpose of pranayama is to evolve the psychic and causal bodies.

Therefore, pranayama sadhana as distinct from general practice may be defined as a concerted, regular and determined effort to achieve perfection in the practice. The goal is not merely good health and mental balance, but acquiring the highest state of consciousness. A dynamic effort must be made to arrive at this state.

While general practitioners may modify a few rules as per convenience (for example, if a separate room is not available for the practice, they may make do with what is available), no slackness in the guidelines is admissible for those wanting to practise pranayama at the level of sadhana. With respect to this aim, the stringent conditions for pranayama sadhana mentioned in the traditional texts assume significance. Strict guidelines for personal conduct

127

are outlined before pranayama instructions are given in *Shiva Samhita* (3:17):

Nabhavetsangayuktaanaam tathaa'vishvaasinaamapi;
Gurupoojaaviheenaanaam tathaa cha bahusanginaam.
Mithyaavaadarataanaam cha tathaa nishthurabhaashinaam;
Gurusantoshaheenaanaam na siddhih syaatkadaachana.

Those who are addicted to sensual pleasures or keep bad company, who are disbelievers, who are devoid of respect towards their guru, who resort to promiscuous assemblies, who are addicted to false and vain controversies, who are cruel in their speech, and who do not give satisfaction to their guru never attain success.

The pranayama sadhaka must improve his or her involvement with life at large and must improve every interaction, whether emotional, intellectual or physical. A state of balance at every level is emphasized time and again for the pranayama practitioner. In Sage Patanjali's *Yoga Sutras*, the practice of pranayama is placed after the practices of yama, niyama and asana. A general practitioner may take to pranayama after shatkarmas and asana, but the sadhaka must overhaul his entire attitude towards life.

Special diets are prescribed during intensive and rigorous pranayama sadhana when the pranic intake through air is amplified and less energy is required through food. Dietary considerations, however, should be obtained from the guru. The *Shiva Samhita* (3:33–37) says the sadhaka must give up foods which are acidic, astringent, pungent, salty and bitter.

One is also advised to take food when the right swara flows and go to sleep when the left swara flows, because pingala is heating and digests the food quickly, whereas ida is cooling and is conducive to calm sleep. Extremes such as fasting, and taking tobacco, cannabis, narcotics and hallucinogenic drugs must be strictly avoided.

The pranayama sadhana must be commenced either in spring or autumn, when the weather is moderate. *Gheranda Samhita* (5:9) says:

Vasante sharadi proktam yogaarambham samaacharet;
Tadaa yogee bhavetsiddho rogaanmukto bhaveddhruvam.

It is correct to start the practices during spring and autumn. When yogic practices are undertaken during these seasons, one certainly attains success and becomes free from diseases.

High mountains and cold climates, where the pure air is thick with negative ions, are most helpful for intensive pranayama sadhana. The yoga texts also state that the pranayama practitioner should not warm himself by fire, because fire depletes negative ions.

The place of practice must be treated as sacred. In *The Yoga Shastra of Dattatreya* (v. 107–111), the place of practice is described:

Sushobhanam matham kuryaatsookshmadvaaram tu nirghunam;
Sushtthu liptam gomayena sudhayaa vaa prayatnatah;
Matkunaih mashakaih bhootaih varjitam cha prayatnatah;
Dine-dine susammrishtham sammaarjanyaa hyatandritah;
Vaasitam cha sugandhena dhoopitam guggulaadibhih.

To practise pranayama, the yogi should prepare a small cloister. The door should be small and the room should be free of all germs. The floor and walls should be wiped carefully with cow dung or lime, so that the room remains free of bugs, mosquitoes and spiders. It should be swept daily and perfumed with incense and resin.

Four sittings of pranayama practice should be undertaken daily at the following times: early morning, midday, evening and midnight. While practising one must sit facing east or north. Nadi shodhana pranayama should be practised for at least three months until the count of 20:80:40:40 is achieved, before commencing any other pranayama.

The sadhaka should avoid excessive company. Sage Dattatreya says, "The pranayama yogi should avoid the company of others and not allow himself to be touched by others." One becomes highly sensitive in the beginning stages of pranayama sadhana and is easily disturbed by external influences. The resulting fluctuations hamper the steadiness of sadhana. Interactions also involve a pranic element. Exchanges that are not uplifting, such as criticism, gossip, or catering to emotional demands, deplete one of prana as well as creating or reinforcing the negative samskaras that one is trying to eliminate through the sadhana. Emotional dependency expressed through an exchange translates into pranic dependency, making it difficult to generate prana as well as remain self-reliant – the two hallmarks of a yogi.

Deep faith in the practice itself is most essential. Only through a commitment born of faith will one be able to continue the practice, irrespective of signs of progress or the inclination to give up when circumstances are unfavourable. *Shiva Samhita* (3:18) says:

> *Phalishyateeti vishvaasah siddheh prathamalakshanaam;*
> *Dviteeya shraddhayaa yuktam triteeyam gurupoojanam.*
> *Chaturtham samataabhaavam panchamendriyanigraham;*
> *Shashtam cha pramitaahaaram saptamam naiva vidyate.*

> The first condition of success is the firm belief that it (vidya) must succeed and be fruitful; the second condition is having faith in it; the third is respect towards the guru; the fourth is the spirit of universal equality; the fifth is the restraint of the organs of sense; the sixth is moderate eating, these are all. There is no seventh condition.

However, even if all the conditions are fulfilled, the sadhaka will not be able to achieve his goal without the grace of guru. The guru and the sadhaka's devotion to him are indispensable when the pranayama practice is taken to the level of sadhana. In *Shiva Samhita* (3:11) it is written:

Bhavedveeryavatee vidyaa guruvaktrasamudbhavaa;
Anyathaa phalaheenaa syaannirveeryaapyatiduhkhadaa.

Only the knowledge imparted by a guru, through his lips, is powerful and useful; otherwise it becomes fruitless, weak and painful.

In pranayama sadhana for the awakening of higher consciousness, the sadhaka prepares to become a channel. Therefore, the guidance of a guru is essential, not just to correct the mechanics of the practice but to transmit intuitive knowledge. With the establishment of a link with the guru, the sadhana becomes the means to receive direction in one's spiritual growth, and the final goal is reached.

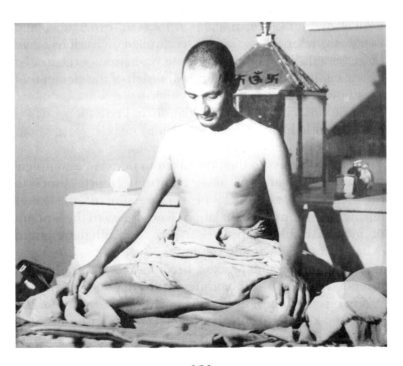

5

Preliminary Breathing Practices

PREPARATION FOR PRANAYAMA

Why is the ability to control the breath a prerequisite for pranayama?

Swami Niranjanananda: Each of the three elements of pranayama – *pooraka*, inhalation, *rechaka*, exhalation, and *kumbhaka*, retention – can be controlled in various ways. More benefit can be obtained from pranayama practices by increasing the degree of control over each of the elements of breathing. Breath control means altering:
• Duration of inhalation, exhalation and retention
• Depth of inhalation and exhalation
• Force of inhalation and exhalation.

Duration refers to the time taken to perform a complete inhalation, exhalation and retention. Depth refers to the degree of expansion or compression of the lungs duringinhalation and exhalation. Force refers to the amount of muscular effort applied to produce inhalation and exhalation or to maintain retention.

As the pranayama practice becomes more advanced, an extended duration of breathing and retention is required. It is necessary to progress comfortably, without strain or the need to take interim breaths. Hence, along with duration, the depth of breathing should be increased in order to meet

132

oxygen requirements. At the same time, the force of the breath should be correspondingly minimized to decrease oxygen consumption and tension in the body. Specific techniques are suggested to gradually extend breathing capacity.

When should deep breathing be practised?

Swami Niranjanananda: The practice of deep breathing should be performed for a few minutes daily in the fresh air of early morning. Each deep breath consists of a full inhalation and a long steady exhalation through the nose. The breath should be inhaled and exhaled slowly to full capacity.

What is viloma pranayama (reverse breath)?

Swami Niranjanananda: In viloma pranayama the breathing is interrupted throughout inhalation and/or exhalation. In normal breathing, inhalation and exhalation flow smoothly and evenly. *Viloma*, meaning 'opposite', here indicates interruption of the natural flow of breath. This practice develops control over the breath flow and is an easy method of extending the breath duration. It may be used as a preparation for nadi shodhana and bhastrika.

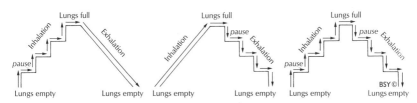

Viloma pranyama, Techniques 1–3

What is rhythmic breathing?

Swami Niranjanananda: Rhythmic breathing techniques induce conscious control of the breathing rhythm. They are all based on equalizing the duration of inhalation and exhalation (1:1 ratio).

133

The breathing rhythm is never constant, but continually changes in response to the demands placed upon the body and mind. During different activities, such as sleeping, eating, walking, riding a bicycle or reading, the rhythm and duration of the breath vary. Different mental states are also reflected in the breathing pattern. Throughout the day the rhythm of the breath is constantly changing, usually without one's knowledge. Rhythmic breathing produces a calming effect and can be used to stabilize the mind during periods of tension and turmoil. Both body and mind respond positively to rhythmic breathing.

What is the purpose of extending the exhalation in pranayama?

Swami Niranjanananda: Inhalation is an active movement, whereas exhalation is a passive movement of relaxation, a state of repose. The heart beats more slowly during exhalation than during inhalation. By slowly lengthening the exhalation, the state of relaxation arises, bringing many benefits to the physical and mental levels. While extending the exhalation, the abdominal muscles are contracted, which has a strengthening effect. Extended exhalation also lessens pain, as in crying and sobbing, which produce slightly extended bursts of exhalation. This is nature's way of dulling pain, both physical and mental. Regular practice of extended exhalation will help in times of stress, as well as in the performance of classical pranayama with advanced ratios.

What is kumbhaka?

Swami Niranjanananda: There are three types of breath retention: *antaranga kumbhaka* or internal retention, *bahiranga kumbhaka* or external retention, and *kevala kumbhaka* or spontaneous retention. The last occurs when the breath automatically ceases and no effort is applied.

Kumbhaka exists in normal respiration, but only for a split second and it is not conscious or controlled. Several preliminary practices are taught to help one develop the awareness of kumbhaka, so that it is familiar when required in the pranayama techniques. Each stage should be mastered before proceeding to the next.

What precautions should be followed when practising kumbhaka?

Swami Niranjanananda: Seek competent guidance before attempting the practices of kumbhaka. These techniques should be approached slowly, moving systematically and comfortably through each stage.

Kumbhaka should not be practised by people with high blood pressure, cardiovascular problems, vertigo, cerebral diseases and mental defects.

The preliminary techniques of inhalation, exhalation and rhythmic breathing should be perfected before starting internal retention. Again, internal retention should be mastered before proceeding to external retention. If the body or mind feels tense in any way, it means that one's natural capacity has been exceeded. One should then stop and go back to the previous stage. By practising slowly, the foundation will be solid.

What is samavritti pranayama?

Swami Niranjanananda: The word *sama* means 'equal', 'even' or 'perfect'; *vritti* literally means 'movement' or 'action'. Therefore, *samavritti pranayama* is known as the equalizing breath.

In samavritti pranayama the respiration is divided into four equal parts. The inhalation, internal retention, exhalation and external retention are of equal duration, making the ratio 1:1:1:1. This practice produces an even and rhythmic flow of breath. However, external retention is difficult to master. The practitioner should be aware of any internal signals arising during the practice, and release any tension forming in the body or mind before continuing the next round.

Mastery of samavritti pranayama enables one to undertake the classical pranayama practices.

When should one proceed to the next stage of a breathing technique?

Swami Niranjanananda: The preliminary breathing techniques should not involve any strain. If the practitioner feels shortness of breath, dizziness or fainting, he should stop the practice and consult a yoga teacher. The breath should not become overextended at any stage of the practices. The need to take extra breaths during or at the end of the round indicates that the practitioner is overextending his capacity and should go back to a previous stage that feels more comfortable.

The breathing capacity extends slowly with practice. The ratio should be increased weekly or monthly, giving the lungs and muscles time to adapt to each stage. The practitioner should not proceed to a further stage until he can perform the present stage comfortably.

THE SUBTLE BREATH

What is meant by awareness of the subtle breath?

Swami Niranjanananda: Yoga is a science and pranayama is an application of this science. The breathing techniques alone, as a purely mechanical operation, create an appropriate effect on the body, mind and spirit. However, it has been observed that the effect of these techniques can be greatly amplified when they are applied with sensitivity and awareness of their subtle influences, and with a deeper understanding of the relationship between the body, energy and mind. Application of a technique without awareness will produce results; however, the process becomes more efficient with awareness, and the inner knowledge begins to awaken.

By developing sensitivity towards the breath from the gross to the subtle levels, one understands the secrets of the intimate relationships in the cycles of life. Once this knowledge awakens, self-mastery follows. In daily life most things are mechanical and automatic. One eats, works and plays, experiences anger, jealousy and joy, without awareness of what one is doing or feeling. This lack of awareness is carried over into the yogic sadhana. Many practitioners perform as many practices as possible in the allotted time, so that they can finish in time for breakfast. But what do they accomplish? Where is the awareness?

There are certain techniques for increasing sensitivity to the subtle levels of the breath, the flows of swara and the pancha pranas. These practices are intended to awaken an insight into the aspects of breath, prana, body and mind, which are normally beyond the mundane awareness. Although they may be regarded as preliminary techniques, they can also be practised at any level of sadhana.

What is meant by awareness of the swara?
Swami Niranjanananda: *Swara* is the flow of breath in the nostrils. One can easily know which nostril is flowing by blocking one nostril at a time, and observing which flow is stronger. A detailed examination of the breath in the nostrils will give quite specific information about one's psycho-physiological state. The aspects to be examined include:
• Predominance of either the right or left nostril
• Distance the breath extends beyond the nostrils
• Direction in which the breath flows into and out of the nostrils.

Observation of the swara using certain techniques shows that these three aspects are quite variable. When the swara is observed over a long period, it will yield a wealth of information. These techniques can be practised at any time and during any situation.

It is suggested that the swara be observed throughout a range of activities and experiences: for example, sitting, eating, talking, walking, exercising, working, relaxing, meditating, feeling anger, sorrow, happiness, depression,

137

exhilaration, contentment, stress and so on. The breath may be checked before, during and after each of these situations. The practitioner should relate his observations to what he already knows about the ida/pingala system, various tattwas and the pancha pranas. This can become a very involved sadhana in itself.

Why and how do yogis manipulate the swara?

Swami Niranjanananda: During the natural oscillation of the breath between the left and right nostrils, relating to ida and pingala nadis, a balanced flow through both nostrils exists only for a matter of minutes. However, this period of balance can be extended by altering the breath in the nostrils, so that they remain equalized. Particular techniques exist to influence the breath flow to bring about this balance. Alternatively, these practices may be used to increase the flow of breath in either nostril, depending on whether one requires more vital energy (right nostril) or mental energy (left nostril). Methods for altering the swara include *padadhirasana*, the breath balancing pose and *danda kriya*, the stick action.

The body and mind have their own self-regulating mechanisms. One should not assume that because one works at a desk all day, the left nostril should remain dominant during that time. Sometimes, however, one

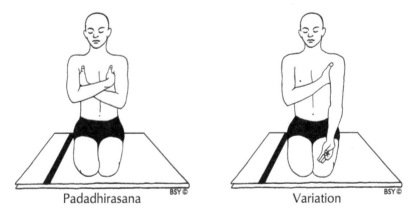

Padadhirasana   Variation

becomes locked into a state of ongoing mental turmoil (left nostril), or competition and aggression (right nostril). At such times, these techniques may be used to change the dominant swara and divert the energies.

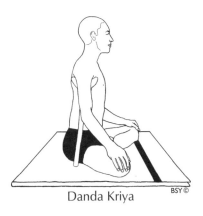
Danda Kriya

These methods are most commonly applied during spiritual practice to maintain a balanced flow in sushumna. At the time of sunrise and sunset either the left or right nostril becomes dominant, depending on the phase of the moon. This is a time of intense swara activity and it is not advised to alter the flows during this period.

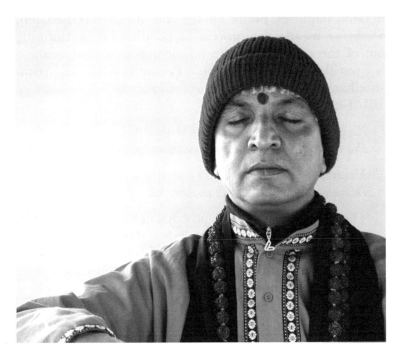

139

6

Nadi Shodhana:
Purification of the Nadis

ABOUT NADI SHODHANA

What is the meaning of the term 'nadi shodhana'?

Swami Satyananda: The most important pranayama is nadi shodhana. The nadis form a network of energy carrying channels. They are physical, vital and psychic, carrying nervous impulses, pranic energy and thoughts respectively. *Shodhana* means the process of purification or throwing out of the toxins and harmful elements. So the meaning is, 'purification of the nadis'. Purification through nadi shodhana is described in *Yoga Chudamani Upanishad* (v. 101–102):

Rechakah poorakashchaiva kumbhakah pranava aatmakah;
Praanaayaamo bhavedevam maatraadvaadashasamyutah.

Maatraadvaadashasamyuktau nishaakara divaakarau;
Doshajaalam abadhnantau jnaatavyau yogibhih sadaa.

The inhalation, retention and exhalation are the Pranava (mantra *Om)* itself. Pranayama should be practised like this for twelve rounds. Twelve rounds through the ida and pingala nadis unfastens the net of impurities. The yogis should know this always. (101–102)

How can the nadis be purified?

Swami Sivananda: Having become firm in the posture and having preserved perfect self-control, the yogi should, in order to clear away the impurities of the sushumna, sit in padmasana, and having inhaled air through the left nostril, retain it as long as he can, and then exhale through the right. Drawing it in again through the right and retaining it, he should then exhale through the left.

To those who practise it according to these rules, through the right and left nostrils, the nadis become purified within three months. He should practise cessation of breath at sunrise, at midday, at sunset and at midnight, slowly, eighty times a day, for four weeks. In the early stage, perspiration is produced; in the middle stage there is tremor of the body; and in the last stage, levitation in the air. These results ensue out of the repression of the breath while sitting in the lotus posture.

When perspiration arises from the effort, one should rub the body well. By this, the body becomes firm and light. In the early course of practice, food with milk and ghee is excellent. Sticking to this rule, one becomes firm in practice and gets no *tapa*, burning sensation, in the body. As lions, elephants and tigers are gradually tamed, so also the breath, when rigidly managed, comes under control.

How is nadi shodhana described in the classical yoga texts?

Swami Niranjanananda: The classical yogic texts all describe nadi purification as a necessary step to achieve *kevala kumbhaka*, spontaneous retention of breath. Many equate pranayama with kumbhaka, while others explain the process to achieve kumbhaka as pranayama. In the first case, nadi shodhana is treated as an indispensable preliminary practice of 'pranayama' and in the second as the first pranayama, or even the only pranayama.

The *Gheranda Samhita* says (5:34):

141

Gheranda uvaacha:
Malaakulaasu naadeeshu maaruto naiva gachchhati;
Praanaayaamah katham siddhyettattvajnaanam katham bhavet;
Tasmaannaadeeshuddhimaadau praanaayaamam tato'bhyaset.

Sage Gheranda replied: If air cannot flow through the
nadis because they are full of waste products, how can
pranayama be perfected, and how can tattwa jnana
(subtle knowledge) manifest?

This implies that first the nadis should be purified, and
then pranayama should be practised. The *Gheranda Samhita*
also recommends the practices of shatkarma and three
specific forms of nadi shodhana, combining bija mantras
and tattwa sadhana to achieve such purification. Thereafter,
it says, "sitting firmly in a posture, let him begin regular
pranayama" (5:36). Among the 'regular pranayamas', the
first is *sahita* – alternate nostril breathing or nadi shodhana
(with or without mantra and visualization), achieving higher
ratios of inhalation, retention and exhalation over a period
of practice.

   In the *Hatha Yoga Pradipika* (2:5) it says:

Shuddhimeti yadaa sarvam naadeechakram malaakulam;
Tadaiva jaayate yogee praanasangrahane kshamah.

When all the nadis and chakras which are full of
impurities are purified, then the yogi is able to retain
prana.

This text treats nadi shodhana as a practice separate
from, and a prelude to, all other pranayamas. It describes
the traditional form of nadi shodhana – alternate nostril
breathing with internal retention, and recommends that it be
practised four times a day, gradually increasing the retention
to eighty counts.

   Sage Dattatreya's *Yoga Shastra* equates pranayama with
the practice of nadi shodhana and lists this pranayama alone,
describing its successive higher stages. He recommends that in

the beginning one should practise four times a day for twenty counts with retention to the best of one's ability. If practised in this way for three months, it will purify all the nadis. In Sage Dattatreya's *Yoga Shastra* it is written (v. 131–132):

Kuryaadevam chaturvaaramanaalasyo dine dine.
Evam maasatrayam kuryaannaadeeshuddhistato bhavet.

This (nadi shodhana) should be performed four times a day every day without sloth. This will bring about nadi shuddhi in three months.

The same assertion has been made in the *Shiva Samhita* and the signs of nadi purification are described in (3:29):

Samakaayah sugandhishcha sukaantih svarasaadhakah;
Aarambhaghatakashchaiva yathaa parichayastadaa;
Nishpattih sarvayogeshu yogaavasthaa bhavanti taah.

The body of the person practising the regulation of breath becomes harmoniously developed, emits sweet scent, and looks beautiful and lovely.

Sage Dattatreya's *Yoga Shastra* ascribes the attributes of a light, bright, lean and thin body to nadi purification. However, to achieve this, the texts say that discipline and balance in food, cravings, sensory experiences, physical activity, company, thought, behaviour and speech are essential along with the practice. If all the rules are followed, nadi purification itself leads the practitioner to experience kevala kumbhaka for as long as desired.

Acquisition of various *siddhis*, psychic powers, may also result, but the practitioner is warned against their influence, and recommended to chant Pranava (the mantra *Om*) to get rid of the associated negative samskaras. This is only the first stage, *arambha avastha*, of kevala kumbhaka, and if the practice of nadi shodhana is continued, the second stage, *ghata avastha*, takes place. This is described in the *Yoga Shastra of Dattatreya* (v. 178–180):

Praanaapaanau manovaayoo jeevaatmaparamaatmanau;
Anyonyasyaavirodhena ekataam ghatato yadaa;
Tadaa ghataadvayaasthaa prasiddhaa yoginaam smritaa.

When the unity of prana and apana, manas and
prana, and atman and paramatman is attained,
and their distinctness removed, this stage is called
ghatadvayavastha or ghatavastha, for which a regular
practice of restraining and sustaining prana is essential.
This stage is known by yogis only.

At this stage, the yogi may practise the pranayama only once
a day. This leads to *pratyahara*, described by Sage Dattatreya
as a practice where sensory withdrawal has been perfected
to the extent that the yogi feels that whatever he sees, hears,
smells, tastes or touches is the Supreme. The *Shiva Samhita*
describes it as a stage where the yogi can hold the breath
for three hours. The third stage, *parichayavastha*, comes only
after the yogi has mastered ghata avastha. In the *Yoga Shastra
of Dattatreya* (v. 212–215):

Tatah parichayaavasthaa jaayate'bhyaasayogatah;
Vaayuh samprerito yatnaadagninaa saha kundaleem;
Bodhayitvaa sushumnaayaam pravishedavirodhatah;
Vaayunaa saha chittam tu pravishechcha mahaapatham.

The stage of parichayavastha comes thereafter if the yogi
continues the yoga practice. The prana, acquainted with
internal fire, awakens the kundalini and enters without
obstacle into the sushumna nadi; the mind also enters
into the great path with the prana.

The aim of pranayama having been achieved, thereafter the
practices of pancha dharana, dhyana and finally, samadhi, are
perfected and nishpatti avastha is attained. Swami Sivananda
states, "A yogic student will automatically experience all these
avasthas one by one, as he advances in his systematic, regular
practices. An impatient student cannot experience any of
these avasthas through occasional practices."

Why is nadi shodhana categorized as a balancing prana-yama?

Swami Niranjanananda: Nadi shodhana is truly a balancing pranayama as whether the imbalance lies in the physical or mental body, it is a practice that can restore equilibrium. Nadi shodhana is practised by alternating the inhalation and exhalation between the left and right nostrils, thus influencing the ida and pingala nadis and the two brain hemispheres. This leads to control of the oscillations of the body-mind network, bringing balance and harmony throughout the system. Nadi shodhana is described in *Shiva Samhita* (3:22–23):

> *Tatashcha dakshaangushthena niruddhya pingalaam sudheeh;*
> *Idayaa poorayedvaayum yathaashaktyaa tu kumbhayet;*
> *Tatastyaktvaa pingalayaashanaireva na vegatah.*

> *Punah pingalayaa"poorya yathaashaktyaa tu kumbhayet;*
> *Idayaa rechayedvaayum na vegena shanaihshanaih.*

> Then let the wise practitioner close with his right thumb the pingala (right nostril), inspire air through the ida (left nostril) and keep the air confined – suspend the breathing – as long as he can; and afterwards let him breathe out slowly, and not forcibly, through the right nostril. (22)

> Again, let him draw breath through the right nostril, and stop breathing as long as his strength permits; then let him expel the air through the left nostril, not forcibly, but slowly and gently. (23)

Why does nadi shodhana have a balancing effect on the brain?

Swami Niranjanananda: The alternate nostril breathing technique used in nadi shodhana pranayama affects the brain hemispheres by alternately stimulating the right brain and then the left brain. The flow of breath through each nostril stimulates the opposite side of the brain via nerve endings just beneath the mucous layer inside the nostrils. Each side of the body is governed by nerves originating in the opposite side of the brain. The stimulation of the nostrils by the flow of breath increases nervous activity in the opposite brain hemisphere.

GUIDELINES FOR PRACTICE

Why does the practice of nadi shodhana start by inhaling through the left nostril?
Swami Niranjanananda: Nadi shodhana, and pranayama generally, are practised to bring the mind under control, and for this purpose the round is usually begun from the left nostril, which represents ida nadi or the mental energy. This activates the right lobe of the brain, which is the intuitive, creative side. The right nostril, which is connected with the left lobe, is the worldly side. In *Hatha Yoga Pradipika* (2:10) it is said:

> *Praanam pibedidayaa pibenniyamitam bhooyo'nyayaa rechayet;*
> *Peetvaa pingalayaa sameeranamatho baddhvaa tyajedvaamayaa.*
> *Sooryaachandramasoranena vidhinaabhyaasam sadaa tanvataam;*
> *Shuddhaa naadiganaa bhavanti yaminaam*
> *maasatrayaadoordhvatah.*

> When the prana is inhaled through the left nostril, then it must be exhaled through the other. When it is inhaled through the right, hold it inside and then exhale through the other nostril. The yami who practises in this way, through the right and left nostrils, alternately purifies all his nadis within three months.

However, if one side is blocked start the practice with whichever nostril is open and clear. If the right is open and clear, begin with the right; if the left is open and clear, begin with the left. If both are blocked or both are open, begin with the left.

146

Why are the early stages of nadi shodhana important?

Swami Satyananda: The early stages of nadi shodhana are essential to prepare the lungs and the nervous system for the following stages, which include breath retention. Unless one develops the ability to breathe slowly and with control, breath retention as practised in pranayama is impossible. It is easy to hold the breath once, but to hold the breath a number of times successively with intermittent inhalations and exhalations requires practice. This is one of the functions of the first stages of nadi shodhana: to prepare the body for the higher practices involving breath retention.

During pranayama practice, try to reduce the movement of the breath to a minimum and increase the duration of breathing to the maximum. If there is any gasping or restlessness or exhaustion, the breath is being forced, and the ratio and counting should be reduced. Pranayama must be developed slowly and systematically so that the lungs and nervous system are never harmed. That is why it is always recommended that pranayama only be practised under the guidance of a teacher or guru.

How does nadi shodhana pranayama work?

Swami Satyananda: According to the yogic concept, the body is fine-tuned to absorb the prana shakti by wilfully lengthening the inhalation and exhalation, and by creating a synchronicity of inhalation and exhalation. This becomes evident when the different stages of nadi shodhana pranayama are studied. First one is taught to simply become aware of the breath, so that breathing is not an unconscious process. In order to create synchronicity of breath, there has to be consciousness of the breathing process.

After that, the process is learning to lengthen inhalation and exhalation by incorporating a ratio. The final ratio of the breath is twenty-four *matras* or counts: inhaling twenty-four counts, exhaling twenty-four counts, which is the length of the *Gayatri* mantra. Yogic texts say, "Breathe in one

Gayatri, retain four *Gayatris* and breathe out two *Gayatris.*" This kind of instruction in yogic literature indicates the number of matras in a mantra. Nadi shodhana has been perfected and complete mastery over the breathing process has been attained when 1:4:2:2 *Gayatri* is perfected. That is twenty-four matras for inhalation multiplied by four times for internal retention, multiplied by two times for both exhalation and external retention.

Of course, people are not used to controlling or regulating the breath, but it is attainable. Even in normal times, if one just breathes in one *Gayatri* and out one *Gayatri,* then in one minute three to five breaths will have been taken. Perfection in pranayama is decided by the ratio and the synchronicity of breath at the time of inhalation and exhalation.

Nadi shodhana becomes effective when one is able to breathe in and out to the same count. Just closing the nostril and opening it will not help as that is just the normal breath. The normal inhalation is always shorter than the exhalation. When the length of the breath is regulated, the entire nervous system associated with the respiratory system is being changed. After all, even in the respiratory system there are nerves which are responsible for the expulsion of air and the intake of air. If a certain rhythm or beat is maintained for breathing in and breathing out, then these nerves inside the lungs and nostrils have to change their natural rhythm and adopt a different one: this different beat helps create a change.

Once this pattern can be followed, a rhythm is created in the respiratory system. This rhythm then creates its own electrical vitality inside the body, much like static energy. If the hands are rubbed together they create static electricity. Similarly, when one breathes in and out in a synchronized manner, this synchronicity affects the flow of ida and pingala. When ida and pingala are totally synchronized with each other, they tend to generate static energy in the physical body and that becomes the first step in the awakening of prana shakti.

148

What method is used to count durations of breaths and retentions in nadi shodhana?

Swami Satyananda: The timing of one matra or count is very important. Today a metronome can be used, but traditionally there were four ways to judge the time: 1. the time taken to circle the knee and snap the fingers; 2. the time taken to clap the hands three times; 3. the time taken for the breath to go in and out while in deep sleep; 4. the time taken to chant *Om*. Of course, during pranayama practice it is not practical to snap the fingers, etc. Counting has to be done mentally in a calm manner – one, *Om*, two, *Om*, three, *Om* . . .

How can the memory and concentration capacity of the brain be increased?

Swami Niranjanananda: To increase the brain capacity nadi shodhana has to be done in a specific way. First of all, imagine a staircase. If a staircase is looked at from the side, one sees the steps. The breath must be coordinated as if one is climbing the steps. For example, if one has to climb seven steps in one breath, visualize breathing in and step up, hold the breath, breathe in, step up, hold the breath, breathe in, step up, etc. This breaks one inhalation into seven steps. Then breathe out in the same manner, so the exhalation is also in seven steps.

First close the right nostril. Breathe in a little – hold – breathe in a little – hold – and like this take seven steps in one breath. Then breathe out and come down the seven steps in the same way. Now, close the left nostril, open the right nostril, and again breathe in – hold – breathe in – hold – for a total of seven steps. Then breathe out and come all the way down the seven steps in the same way.

If there is any feeling of strain, reduce the number of steps. Repeat the same pattern about five times with each nostril to complete the practice of nadi shodhana pranayama. This practice will increase the retention capacity of the brain. It enables one to memorize and concentrate with much less effort. To succeed in studies, and to develop control over the mind, this practice is a must.

Can nadi shodhana be practised mentally?

Swami Niranjanananda: Anuloma viloma is a mental adaptation of nadi shodhana pranayama which has a subtle and balancing effect. Simple nadi shodhana is practised without using nasagra mudra, but with the help of the mind and imagination. This technique subtly demonstrates the power of the mind. Even though one may be imagining the breath in the alternate nostrils at first, in time one will actually feel the breath moving in the nostrils by mental command.

The advantage of this technique is that it can be practised in one's daily sadhana and at other times as well. It can be done while sitting, lying, standing or walking. Anuloma viloma helps one become centred and increases the awareness.

What are the levels of practice for anuloma viloma (mental nadi shodhana)?

Swami Niranjanananda: Anuloma viloma can be practised as per the beginning and intermediate levels of nadi shodhana. By the time the advanced level is reached, the breathing should be very subtle, and anuloma viloma will become superfluous. Anuloma viloma has a calming effect on the nervous system, and can be practised during stressful situations without other people's knowledge. It is an on-the-spot tranquillizer, which also promotes clarity of mind and awareness, without adverse side effects.

Which pranayama should students and children practise?

Swami Satyananda: There are over thirty types of pranayama, but one in particular is good for students and for children. This is known as nadi shodhana.

NADI SHODHANA SADHANA

Which pranayamas are most important for daily practice?

Swami Niranjanananda: Two pranayamas must be practised: nadi shodhana and bhramari. Nadi shodhana balances the two brain hemispheres and removes nervous tensions. Bhramari regulates the functions of the endocrine system. When the functions of the glandular system are regulated and the brain is charged with oxygen and prana shakti, and its two hemispheres are working in coordination, there is a manifold increase in the efficiency of the brain and mind.

What makes nadi shodhana a complete practice in itself?

Swami Niranjanananda: Nadi shodhana is a complete practice in itself; as stated in the scriptures, it can lead to the experience of kevala kumbhaka and samadhi. However, the diligence of a sadhaka is required to arrive at this state. In texts such as *Shiva Samhita,* the various remarkable stages following the practice of nadi shodhana presume such a calibre of aspirant. These scriptures were written by highly accomplished yogis who actually described their own advanced practices. Nevertheless, the practice of nadi shodhana gives substantial benefits to an average practitioner as well. Mastery of nadi shodhana is described in *Yoga Chudamani Upanishad* (v. 99):

> *Yatheshta dhaaranam vaayoranalasya pradeepanam;*
> *Naadaabhivyaktih aarogyam jaayate naadishodhanaat.*

> With full retention of the breath, there is activation of the fire and inner sound is heard. Good health is gained by purification of the nadis.

Swami Satyananda has said of nadi shodhana, "If one wants to lead a spiritual life, this very pranayama is sufficient. It will steady the way to meditation and samadhi."

How long does it take to purify the nadis by the practice of nadi shodhana?

Swami Satyananda: If boils, pimples, diarrhoea, constipation or fever occur, it is most likely due to the nadis rebalancing and purifying themselves. However, one should always check that the lifestyle and diet are suitably balanced and regular, and that one's asana practice is systematic. In *Shiva Samhita* (3:26) it says:

> *Ittham maasatrayam kuryaadanaalasyo dine dine;*
> *Tato naadeevishuddhih syaadavilambena nishchitam.*

> When this (nadi shodhana to twenty counts four times a day) has been practised daily for three months with regularity, the nadis of the body will surely be purified without delay.

Of course, other conditions have to be met for this to take place. One would need to practise regularly for extended periods, devoting many hours to the practice of pranayama only, in order to beneficially practise the higher ratios. Perhaps if the final stage of nadi shodhana with the ratio 20:80:40:60 were practised, the nadis would be purified within three months. For most people, however, it takes longer. Also, if the practitioner reverts to an indulgent lifestyle, the nadis will again become impure. Certain disciplines have to be maintained until the kundalini is awakened, otherwise old conditions will recur.

How can nadi shodhana be used in daily life and for spiritual awakening?

Swami Niranjanananda: As a daily practice, nadi shodhana may be used to vitalize the pranic energies, release pranic blockages and achieve a balance between the sympathetic and parasympathetic nervous systems, so that life's situations can be handled better. As a therapeutic tool, it can be applied for almost all physical and mental disorders, although this must be done under expert guidance. For those

152

who wish to use nadi shodhana as a spiritual practice, it may indeed awaken the dormant shakti and direct it through sushumna, the path of spiritual awakening, leading to deep states of meditation.

How should the practice of nadi shodhana be developed from beginners to advanced?

Swami Niranjanananda: The practice is presented in three parts, beginners, intermediate and advanced. Proper advice should be obtained before commencing any of these levels. As with all techniques, each stage should be mastered before proceeding to the next, so that the duration of inhalation, exhalation and retention can be controlled without strain and without the need to take extra breaths in between rounds.

One should not be alarmed by the long ratios of the advanced level. They are difficult to master and are intended only for the serious sadhaka. The practitioner who becomes competent in all the stages of beginner and intermediate levels will gain the full benefit of the practice, physically, mentally and spiritually. Progress beyond this point is sadhana to be undertaken only under the strict guidance of a master. Guidelines for advanced sadhana of nadi shodhana are described in *Shiva Samhita* (3:24–25):

Idam yogavidhaanena kuryaadvimshatikumbhakaan;
Sarvadvandvavinirmuktah pratyaham vigataalasah.

Praatahkaale cha madhyaahne sooryaaste chaarddharaatrake;
Kuryaadevam chaturvaaram kaaleshveteshu kumbhakaan.

According to the above method of yoga, let him practise twenty kumbhakas (stopping of the breath). He should practise this daily without neglect or idleness, and free from all dualities (of love and hatred, and doubt and contention), etc. (24)

These kumbhakas should be practised four times: once early in the morning at sunrise, then at midday, the third at sunset and the fourth at midnight. (25)

153

What should the duration of nadi shodhana pranayama be for the average practitioner?

Swami Satyananda: Nadi shodhana pranayama is so effective that it only has to be done for about ten minutes every morning; not even ten, five will suffice. Simply breathe in through the left nostril slowly, hold the breath in for about two seconds, breathe out through the right nostril, then breathe in through the right nostril, retain for two seconds, and breathe out through the left nostril. This is done in a continuous flow and constitutes one round. In this way five rounds can easily be practised each morning, increasing the number as one feels ready to, up to ten or twenty rounds. Nadi shodhana is described in the *Yoga Chudamani Upanishad* (v. 98):

> *Praanam chedidayaa pibenniyamitam bhooyoh anyathaa rechayet;*
> *Peetvaa pingalayaa sameeranamatho baddhvaa tyadjedvaamayaa;*
> *Sooryaachandramasoranena vidhinaa bindudvayaṁ dhaayatah;*
> *Shuddha naadiganaa bhavanti yamino maasadvayaadoordhvatah.*

The breath should be drawn in through the left nostril, retained and taken out through the right. Again, the breath should be drawn in through the right and retained, then taken out through the left. By practising this method regularly, one gains control over both points of sun and moon, and the energy channels become purified within two months.

How can mantra repetition be used in conjunction with nadi shodhana?

Swami Satyananda: When pranayama is performed without repetition of mantra it is known as *nirgarbha*. When mantra is repeated with inhalation, exhalation and retention, it is known as *sagarbha*. The method of sagarbha nadi shodhana given in the *Gheranda Samhita* (5:38–42) is:

> *Vaayubeejam tato dhyaatvaa dhoomravarnam satejasam.*
> *Chandrenapooryedvaayum beejam shodashakaih sudheeh;*

Chatuhshashtyaa maatrayaa cha kumbhakenaiva dhaarayet;
Dvaatrimshanmaatrayaa vaayum sooryanaadyaa cha rechayet.

Naabhimoolaadvahnimutthaapya dhaayettejovaneeyutam;

Vahnibeejashodasena sooryanaadyaa cha poorayet.

Chatuhshashtyaa cha maatrayaa kumbhakenaiva dhaarayet;
Dvaatrishanmaatrayaa vaayum shashinaadyaa cha rechayet.

Keeping in mind the vayu bija mantra *Yam*, inhale through the left nostril (chandra marga), repeating the bija mantra sixteen times. In the meditative state one should consider this vayu bija to be the colour of bright smoke. Thus after inhalation through the left nostril, one should perform kumbhaka (holding the breath), repeating the mantra sixty-four times, and then repeating it thirty-two times perform exhalation through the right nostril. (38–39)

Raise the fire element (agni tattwa) from the navel centre and meditate on its light associated with earth. Keeping in mind the *Ram* bija and repeating this mantra sixteen times one should inhale through the right nostril (surya nadi), perform kumbhaka while repeating it up to sixty-four times and then exhale through the left nostril, repeating the mantra thirty-two times. (40–42)

This is the traditional method and there are variations. Sage Gheranda continues (5:43–44):

Naasaagre shashadhrigbimbam dhyaatvaa jyotsnaasamanvitam;
Tham beeja shodashenaiva idayaa poorayenmarut.

Chatuhshashtyaa maatrayaa cha vam beejenaiva dhaarayet;
Amritam plaavitam dhyaatvaa naadeedhautim vibhaavayet;
Dvaatrimshena lakaarena dridham bhaavyam virechayet.

Focus the mind on the image of the moon at the nosetip and repeat the bija manta *Tham* sixteen times while inhaling through the left nostril. (43)

One should retain the breath in sushumna, repeating the bija mantra *Vam* 64 times. One should fix the mind on the flow of nectar from the moon at the tip of the nose and clean all the nadis with it. Then one should exhale through the right nostril by repeating the *Lam* bija mantra thirty-two times. (44)

This is a ratio of 1:4:2. However, such high proportions are unnecessary for general use. The ratio should be adjusted to individual capacity.

PREPARATION FOR HIGHER PRACTICE

Why is nadi shodhana an important preparation for other pranayamas?

Swami Niranjanananda: Nadi shodhana is the first pranayama described in the classical yogic texts. Ideally, other classical pranayamas should be attempted only after practising nadi shodhana as instructed by the teacher for a specific period. The word *nadi* means 'energy channel' and *shodhana* means 'to cleanse' or 'to purify'. Therefore, *nadi shodhana* is a practice whereby the pranic channels are purified and regulated. This prepares one for the practice of other pranayamas, so that maximum benefits can be derived and one does not experience any pranic imbalance. In *Hatharatnavali* (3:82) it is written:

Malaakulaasu naadeeshu maaruto naiva madhyagah;
Katham syaadunmaneebhaavah kaaryasiddhih katham bhavet.

If the nadis are full of impurities, Maruta (the god of wind i.e. prana) does not travel along the middle path (sushumna nadi). How then can one attain the state of unmani? How can one succeed in one's aim?

What are the mental and spiritual effects of nadi shodhana?

Swami Niranjanananda: Nadi shodhana activates the frontal brain and ajna chakra, thereby inducing tranquillity, clarity of thought and concentration. It also helps remove depressive tendencies. At the spiritual level, the practice of nadi shodhana prepares one to enter higher meditative states.

Is nadi shodhana useful before meditation?

Swami Satyananda: Nadi shodhana with a ratio of 1:1 is most effective for balancing the air flow through the two nostrils. For this reason it is particularly useful before relaxation and meditation techniques. It develops a state of harmony in the individual so that he is neither too lethargic nor too active, too dull or too excitable. The pranic currents, or poles of ida and pingala, moon and sun, are brought into balance with each other, increasing the health of the whole body-mind complex.

How does nadi shodhana prepare one for dharana?

Swami Satyananda: The ratio is important in pranayama because it is directly linked with the right and left hemispheres of the brain and with the sympathetic and parasympathetic nervous systems. There has to be a ratio in pranayama, not so much for the sake of oxygenation but in order to influence the brain.

The ideal ratio, which will completely put the mind under control so that it can't move, is 1:6:4:4, but one cannot start with this. One must start with the minimum ratio which is 1:2. Later it can be increased to 1:3, 1:4, 1:5, and 1:6. After completing each round of nadi shodhana, the awareness is fixed at the eyebrow centre, and concentration on one's symbol is begun. This is practised for a short time, maybe a minute or two, not more than that, then the second round is started. In between each round, practise concentration. If five rounds of pranayama are practised, then five rounds of concentration will be done.

In the beginning the five rounds will take five minutes, but when one is properly established in the practice, five rounds will take three hours. At that stage, just one round is enough. When this one round of pranayama has been practised, that person is ready to start concentration.

How can pranayama be used to manage the emotions?

Swami Niranjanananda: In the *Bhagavad Gita* Arjuna poses a question. "How do I control passion? You have spoken of antar mouna as the process to manage conditions and states of fear, anxiety and attachments, but how do I manage passions?" Sri Krishna gives Arjuna a sadhana: to fix the mind at the eyebrow centre and regulate the breath, making the inhalation and exhalation as long as possible, and during the gap between inhalation and exhalation, focus the awareness on the inner Self. This is the practice of nadi shodhana pranayama.

By placing the two fingers at the eyebrow centre, a pressure point is created to enable the mind to become fixed at the eyebrow centre. Regulate the breath to a minimum of twenty-four *matras*, units, per incoming and outgoing breath. Each matra is like a second. The *Gayatri* mantra of twenty-four matras is used to practise nadi shodhana pranayama: *Om tatsavitur varenyam bhargo devasya dheemahi dhiyo yo nah prachodayaat.* Twenty-four matras make one inhalation. This is the training that Sri Krishna imparts in the *Bhagavad Gita* (5:27–28) to keep the mind fixed:

Sparshaankritvaa bahirbaahyaamshchakshushchaivaantare bhruvoh;
Praanaapaanau samau kritvaa naasaabhyantarachaarinau.

Yatendriya manobuddhirmunirmokshaparaayanah;
Vigatechchhaabhayakrodho yah sadaa mukta eva sah.

Shutting out (all) external contacts and fixing the gaze between the eyebrows, equalizing the outgoing and incoming breaths moving within the nostrils, with the senses, the mind and the intellect always controlled, having liberation as his supreme goal, free from desire, fear and anger – the sage is verily liberated forever. (27–28)

When the breath is regulated, the brainwaves are affected. High alpha and theta waves predominate, and with these predominating, the nervous system and mental dimension experience a state of relaxation and a balance of energies: physical, sensorial, mental, emotional, psychic and spiritual.

When pranayama is practised slowly, the body feels different, and when pranayama is practised fast, the body feels different: fast pranayama and rapid breathing affect the condition of the body. However, the *Bhagavad Gita* indicates long, deep breathing and lengthening the ratio of breath. Slow and deep breathing relaxes the physical structure, the nervous system and the brain. This relaxed condition in turn influences mental and psychological behaviour. Many therapists use pranayama to create a change in the mental behaviour of mentally unstable people. By balancing the energies of ida and pingala, positive personality changes come about.

Sri Krishna speaks of pranayama as a method of managing the hyperactive and passionate mental behaviours. Passion is not always sensorial, sensual or sexual. Passion is any desire or thought that dominates the mind. It represents a condition of mental behaviour in which one item becomes predominant and highlighted, and all reactions, responses, actions, thoughts and interactions revolve around that one particular thought or idea. This sustained mental function is known as passion, which can be directed and used for anything. An artist can become a passionate artist, a sculptor can become a passionate sculptor, a yogi can become a passionate yogi. That energy, awareness and mentality can take any form and shape, negative or positive, tamasic or sattwic.

By regulating the prana shakti, pranayama balances the extreme behaviour of the passions and levels out the mental extremes. In this way, Sri Krishna teaches ways of managing different types of situations which are encountered on a daily basis by using simple practices of yoga and ideas to cultivate understanding and awareness.

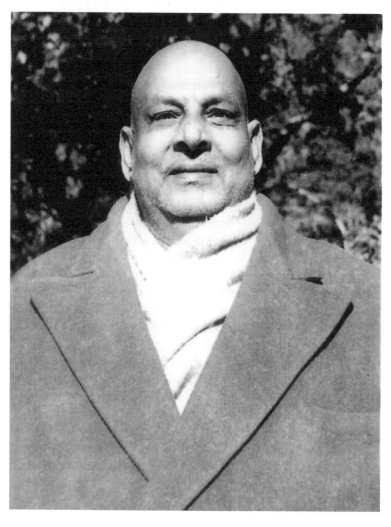

7

Tranquillizing Pranayamas

ABOUT TRANQUILLIZING PRANAYAMAS

What is the purpose of the tranquillizing pranayamas?
Swami Niranjanananda: The tranquillizing practices of pranayama are designed to relax the body and mind while simultaneously increasing the pranic capacity and conscious awareness. These pranayamas stimulate the parasympathetic nervous system and draw the awareness within. Some bring about greater psychic sensitivity, while others cool the system.

When are tranquillizing pranayamas practised?
Swami Niranjanananda: The tranquillizing techniques are usually practised after nadi shodhana, which balances the sympathetic and parasympathetic nervous systems by regulating the flow of breath in the alternate nostrils. Therefore, the tranquillizing practices are done through both nostrils together and in some cases through the mouth.

When should tranquillizing pranayamas be avoided?
Swami Niranjanananda: These practices should be avoided by persons who are excessively introverted, oversensitive or psychically unbalanced, as they may exacerbate these conditions.

161

SHEETKARI PRANAYAMA: HISSING BREATH
AND SHEETALI PRANAYAMA: COOLING BREATH

What is sheetkari pranayama?

Swami Satyananda: In sheetkari pranayama the sound 'shee' or 'sheet' is made during inhalation. The Sanskrit word *kari* means 'that which produces'. The practice produces the sound 'shee' and it also produces coolness.

What are the effects of sheetkari pranayama?

Swami Satyananda: Sheetkari cools the body and should therefore be practised during warm seasons, not in winter unless particularly specified by the guru. If the weather is extremely hot it can be practised for more than ten minutes. In moderate heat, ten to fifteen rounds is sufficient. It is often practiced after bhastrika pranayama, especially if bhastrika is practised during summer, to counterbalance the excess heat produced in the body.

When the breath is drawn in through the mouth, as in this pranayama, it has a cooling effect. Just as an animal pants in the heat to cool the body, when one inhales through the mouth it cools the tongue, oral cavity and throat, therefore the inhaled air is cooler and the cooling effect is also felt in other regions.

This pranayama also has another important effect. When the breath is taken in through the mouth, the nerves in the nose which register the moisture, temperature, ions, etc., in the air are not stimulated, though of course the ions and air are nevertheless absorbed into the body.

In *Hatha Yoga Pradipika* (2:54), Yogi Swatmarama mentions that the practitioner of sheetkari becomes Kamadeva the second:

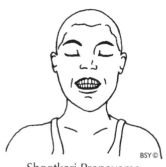

Sheetkari Pranayama

162

Seetkaam kuryaattathaa vaktreghraanenaiva vijrimbhikaam;
Evamabhyaasayogena kaamadevo dviteeyakah.

By drawing the breath in through the mouth, make a hissing sound, without gaping the mouth, and exhale through the nose. By practising this, one becomes a second Kamadeva (god of love).

In Hindu mythology Kamadeva is the god of love and passion. He is something like Cupid and is the personification of sensual desire and affection. Of course this does not mean that sheetkari pranayama makes one lustful, rather it makes the practitioner virile and attractive.

Passion is a form of heat in the body and mind, which in sensual life is expressed and discharged in the natural way. This results in an energy loss. Through sheetkari the mental and emotional inflammation of passion is reduced. One is able to maintain vital energy and control, and have a magnetic and attractive aura.

What are the subtle and esoteric effects of sheetkari pranayama?
Swami Satyananda: *Hatha Yoga Pradipika* (2:55), describes the effects of sheetkari in a mysterious way:

Yoginee chakrasammaanyahsrishtisamhaarakaarakah;
Na kshudhaa na trishaa nidraa naivaalasyam prajaayate.

He is adored by the circle of yoginis and becomes the controller of creation and dissolution, being without hunger, thirst, sleep and laziness.

According to this sloka, the one who perfects sheetkari is adored or worshipped by the chakra or circle of yoginis, but what exactly is the chakra of yogini? *Chakra* usually refers to a particular circle which is a source of energy. A yogini is a female yogi, the embodiment of Shakti, the cosmic, creative force. In tantra there is an order of sixty-four yoginis who represent the sixty-four tantras and the sixty-four perfections of yoga.

The aspects and evolution of cosmic shakti from its source are represented by the Sri yantra which is also called Sri chakra. The *Sri yantra* is the formula of creation, manifestation and dissolution of the macro and microcosmos. It is constituted by a number of interlacing triangles which are known as *yoginis*. They represent the cosmic shakti and manifestation of human existence. Sri yantra also represents each individual.

The chakra of yoginis symbolizes every function of the gross and subtler bodies, the functions of mind, and integration with the soul. Our entire existence is controlled or operated by various forms of shakti represented as a specific yogini or devi. Each individual person is a manifestation of the chakra of yoginis. Thus it is said that through the practice of sheetkari the whole body comes under the control of the practitioner. In fact, perfection of any of the pranayamas leads to control of the body mechanisms, stabilization of the mental tendencies and deeper awareness of the mind-body complex.

Sheetkari particularly works on the aspect of the heat and cold in the body. Control of any two opposite forces in the body-mind leads to control of the other aspects of the physical, mental, emotional and psychic makeup. Yogi Swatmarama specifically mentions that sheetkari eliminates indolence and the need and desire to eat, drink and sleep.

What is the effect of sheetkari on the gunas?
Swami Satyananda: There are three qualities or *gunas* of the body-mind and nature which bind the consciousness: tamas, rajas and sattwa. Each of us has these three qualities but they do not exist in equal proportions, one always predominates. In order to achieve higher states of consciousness, sattwa has to become predominant, although ultimately one must go beyond that.

Most people in this kali yuga are *tamasic* – dull and lethargic, or *rajasic* – dynamic and ambitious by nature, but through yoga and other evolutionary sciences, *sattwa* –

balance, harmony and one-pointedness, can be developed. Sattwa represents the highest point in the evolution of the human mind. *Hatha Yoga Pradipika* (2:56) says that sheetkari leads to sattwa:

Bhavetsattvam cha dehasya sarvopadravavarjitaah;
Anena vidhinaa satyam yogeendro bhoomimandale.

And the sattwa in the body becomes free from all disturbances. Truly, by the aforementioned method one becomes lord of yogis on this earth.

Here, Yogi Swatmarama is saying that through the practice of sheetkari pranayama, the body and mind can both be brought into a state of harmony and thereafter sattwa will become the dominating quality. One who has completely transcended tamas and rajas and is ruled by sattwa, is indeed a great yogi.

What is the difference between sheetkari and sheetali pranayamas?
Swami Satyananda: In the practice of sheetkari the breath is inhaled through the teeth, while in sheetali it is inhaled through the rolled tongue. About one-third of the population is unable to roll the tongue into a tube and will need to use sheetkari.

Sheetali means 'the cooling breath' and it also means calm, passionless, unemotional. Like sheetkari, this pranayama was specifically designed to reduce the body temperature. However, these practices not only cool and calm the physical body, they affect the mind in the same way. Sheetali is described in *Hatha Yoga Pradipika* (2:57):

Jihvayaa vaayumaakrishya poorvavatkumbhasaadhanam;
Shanakairghraanarandhraabhyaam rechayet pavanam sudheeh.

The wise inhale air through the tongue and practise kumbhaka (as described before), then exhale the air through the nostrils.

165

The benefits of sheetali and sheetkari are basically the same. These two practices are unique because inhalation is done through the mouth. In every other yogic practice, and in breathing in general, breathing is through the nose. When the breath is taken through the nose, the nose warms and cleans the incoming air. Therefore, it is important not to practise these pranayamas in a dirty, polluted atmosphere or in excessively cold weather.

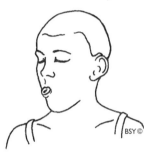

Sheetali Pranayama

There is only a slight difference between sheetkari and sheetali. In sheetkari awareness is focused on the hissing sound and in sheetali it is kept on the cooling sensation of the breath. There are also minor differences which affect different parts of the nervous system, but ultimately the impulses are sent to the central nervous system and brain.

Why are sheekari and sheetali known as cooling breaths?

Swami Satyananda: When one breathes through the teeth or tongue the air is cooled by the saliva and this cools the blood vessels in the mouth, throat and lungs. In turn, the stomach, liver and whole body are cooled. Because sheetali and sheetkari soothe away mental tension, they are useful techniques for alleviating psychosomatic disease such as high blood pressure. They also purify the blood and improve digestion.

How long should breath retention be practised during sheetali?

Swami Niranjanananda: In *Gheranda Samhita* Sage Gheranda's instructions are not to practise *kumbhaka*, breath retention, for as long as possible. Rather there should be an interval of just a moment between inhalation and exhalation. During that momentary breath retention, the tongue is pulled in, the mouth is closed and the breath is expelled through the nose. This makes one round. In *Gheranda Samhita* (5:74) it is written:

Jihvayaa vaayumaakrishya chodare poorayechchhanaih;
Kshanam cha kumbhakam kritvaa naasaabhyaam rechayetpunah.

Fill the abdomen by sucking air through the tongue. Retain the air for a short while with the help of kumbhaka and expel it through both nostrils.

What are the effects of practising sheetali?
Swami Niranjanananda: Sheetali affects important brain centres associated with biological drives and temperature regulation. It reduces body heat and also cools the mind. It reduces blood pressure, acidity in the stomach, and mental and emotional excitation, and encourages the free flow of prana throughout the body. It induces muscular relaxation, mental tranquillity and may be used as a tranquillizer before sleep.

Sheetali gives control over hunger and excessive sweating and thirst during hot weather, and generates a feeling of satisfaction. A person who masters sheetali pranayama experiences a reduction in thirst and remains cool even in the hottest environment. The metabolic rate is reduced. Physical tiredness due to excessive labour does not last long, yet a state of inner tranquillity is maintained for longer periods.

Sage Gheranda says sheetali is a simple yet extremely useful practice, because if yogis always practise it, digestive diseases and disorders of kapha and pitta do not take place. In *Gheranda Samhita* (5:75) it is written:

Sarvadaa saadhayedyogee sheetaleekumbhakam shubham;
Ajeernam kaphapittam cha naiva tasya prajaayate.

This beneficial sheetali pranayama should always be practised. By practising it, digestive disorders and kapha-pitta disorders do not manifest.

What are the benefits of sheetali pranayama?

Swami Satyananda: *Sheetali* literally means 'cooler'. By practising this pranayama a cooling effect is experienced throughout the body. Sheetali purifies the blood and removes high blood pressure. It gives mental and muscular rest. In *Hatha Yoga Pradipika* (2:58) the benefits of sheetali are explained:

> *Gulmapleehaadikan rogaan jvaram pittam kshudhaam trishaam;*
> *Vishaani sheetalee naama kumbhikeyam nihanti hi.*

This kumbhaka called sheetali cures an enlarged stomach or spleen and other related diseases, fever, excess bile, hunger and thirst, and counteracts poisons.

UJJAYI PRANAYAMA: THE PSYCHIC BREATH

What is ujjayi pranayama?

Swami Satyananda: Ujjayi is one of the most important, yet one of the simplest pranayamas. It is a deep breathing practice which induces a meditative state. It is practised by contracting the glottis. If this is done properly, a slight contraction of the abdomen can simultaneously be detected. It is easy for the practitioner to misunderstand this and make a special point of contracting the abdominal muscles, which must not be done. If the glottis is contracted, there is automatically a slight pulling sensation in the abdominal region.

With each breath there should be a continuous sound emitted from the throat. It should not be loud, it should only be audible to oneself. This sound is caused by the friction of the air as it passes through the restriction that has been made in the glottis by the contraction. The sound will be similar to the gentle sound that a baby makes while sleeping. This form of breathing, together with folding the tongue back in khechari mudra, is known as ujjayi pranayama.

When done correctly, ujjayi sounds soft like a cat purring or light snoring. When a healthy child sleeps at night, he always breathes by contracting his glottis, and the breath can be heard in his throat. Ujjayi is perfected by relaxing the breath rather than forcing it. If one concentrates on the throat and relaxes the breath, it will feel as if the breathing is through the throat. Of course the breath goes through the nostrils, but the glottis is contracted so the feeling is stronger in the throat. Ujjayi is described in *Hatha Yoga Pradipika* (2:51–52):

Mukham samyamya naadeebhyaamaakrishya pavanam shanaih;
Yathaa lagati kanthattu hridayaavadhi sasvanam.

Poorvavatkumbhayetpraanam rechayedidayaa tathaa;
Shleshmadoshaharam kanthe dehanalavivardhanam.

Closing the mouth, inhale with control and concentration through ida and pingala, so that the breath is felt from the throat to the heart and produces a sonorous sound. (51)

Do kumbhaka as before and exhale through ida. This removes phlegm from the throat and stimulates the (digestive) fire. (52)

What is meant by 'psychic breathing'?

Swami Satyananda: Ujjayi means 'victorious'; *ujji* is the root which means 'to conquer' or 'acquire by conquest'. In English, ujjayi is known as the 'psychic breath' because of its effect on the mind. However, the practice of psychic breathing begins with the natural breath. The higher stage of this practice is done with ujjayi, which is both deeper and longer. Initially, however, the aspirant merely becomes aware of his natural breathing, a process one goes through about 21,600 times in every 24 hours, whether one is aware of it or not. It is at the rate of 900 cycles per hour, but no-one is aware of it. The only thing that has to be done is to be aware of the breath, to know one is breathing. The word 'psychic' enters into the picture when the awareness and breathing process become one; then it is called psychic breathing.

At first, awareness should only be practised in this way on the natural breath, but later, ujjayi pranayama should be

169

used. Simultaneously a conscious effort is made to quieten the mind. Even if the mind interferes, if it wanders, the effort must be made to keep stopping it from interfering. It is important to have complete control over the process. After breathing 25 to 30 times in this way, a tendency to begin meditation arises. Ujjayi goes on for a few minutes then it tends to stop. Any such interruption of the pranayama must be prevented: one must maintain control. Consciousness must be held exactly at that point.

What are the benefits of ujjayi?

Swami Niranjanananda: Ujjayi is classified as a tranquillizing pranayama and it also has a heating effect on the body. This practice is used in yoga therapy to soothe the nervous system and calm the mind. It has a profoundly relaxing effect at the psychic level. It helps to relieve insomnia and may be practised in shavasana just before sleeping. The basic form, without breath retention or bandhas, slows down the heart rate and is useful for people suffering from high blood pressure.

Ujjayi removes disorders of the *dhatu*, which are the seven constituents of the body: blood, bone, marrow, fat, semen, skin and flesh. With the practice of ujjayi, the practitioner does not suffer from kapha disorders, constipation, dysentery, intestinal ulcers, colds, fever or liver problems.

With the practice of ujjayi, it is said that fear of death and old age disappears. Generally it has been observed that ujjayi is particularly useful in the practice of pratyahara.

In *Gheranda Samhita* (5:72–73) the benefits of ujjayi are given:

Ujjaayee kumbhakam kritvaa sarvakaaryaanisaadhayet;
Na bhavetkapharogashcha krooravaayurajeernakam.

Aamavaatah kshayah kaaso jvarah pleehaa na vidyate;
Jaraamrityuvinaashaaya chojjaayeem saadhayennarah.

This is called ujjayi kumbhaka. With it all works are perfected. Diseases from kapha imbalances, nervous and digestive disorders do not manifest. (72)

Diseases concerning mucus, tuberculosis, respiratory disorders, fever and spleen-related disorders are cured. If ujjayi kumbhaka is perfected, old age and death are also managed. (73)

What precautions should be observed when practising ujjayi?

Swami Niranjanananda: People who are too introverted by nature should not perform this practice. Those suffering from heart disease should not combine bandhas or breath retention with ujjayi.

What posture is best for the practice of ujjayi?

Swami Niranjanananda: Ujjayi may be performed in any position, standing, sitting or lying. Those suffering from slipped disc or vertebral spondylitis may practise ujjayi in vajrasana or makarasana. Many people contort their facial muscles while doing ujjayi. It is unnecessary. Try to relax the face as much as possible.

Can ujjayi be used at any time?

The practice of ujjayi is so simple that it can be done anywhere and in any position. This is stated in *Hatha Yoga Pradipika* (2:53):

Naadeejalodaraadhaatugatadoshavinaashanam;
Gachchhataa tishthataa kaaryamujjaayyaakhyam tu kumbhakam.

This pranayama, called ujjayi, can be done while moving, standing, sitting or walking. It removes dropsy and disorders of the nadis and dhatu.

How does one know if ujjayi is being practised correctly?

Swami Satyananda: It is possible that the practitioner will not be sure if ujjayi is being done correctly. Many people contort their facial muscles when they do ujjayi. This is unnecessary. The face should be relaxed as much as possible and it's important not to overcontract the throat. The contraction should be slight and applied continuously throughout the practice.

A similar contraction of the throat is obtained when one whispers aloud. If one whispers loudly enough for a person a few metres away to hear it, this should help indicate the method of contracting the glottis. However, this is only intended as an illustration and whispering should not be incorporated into ujjayi pranayama.

How does ujjayi pranayama help regulate blood pressure?

Swami Satyananda: In the neck there are two remarkable organs called the carotid sinuses. They are situated on each side of the main artery supplying the brain with blood, in front of the neck and just below the level of the jaws. These small organs help to control and regulate blood flow and pressure. If there is any fall in blood pressure, it is detected by these two sinuses and the relevant message is sent directly to the brain centre. The brain responds immediately by increasing the heartbeat and contracting the arterioles (tiny blood vessels), thus raising the pressure to its normal level. Any rise in blood pressure is also detected by the carotid sinuses, which inform the brain, and the opposite steps are taken to rectify the situation.

Tension and stress are associated with high blood pressure. Ujjayi pranayama, by applying a slight pressure on these sinuses in the neck, causes them to react as though they have detected high blood pressure. The heartbeat and the blood pressure then reduce below normal and one becomes physically and mentally relaxed. This is the reason why ujjayi is important in many meditation practices. It induces overall relaxation, which is essential for success in meditation.

Khechari mudra, the tongue lock, accentuates this pressure in the throat region and consequently on the two carotid sinuses. Anyone can experiment by doing ujjayi firstly without khechari mudra, and then with, comparing the difference in pressure.

Ujjayi pranayama is a simple practice but it has many subtle influences on the body and brain, both physical and mental as well as pranic. The slow, deep breathing results in immediate calmness of the mind and body, and also brings the pranic body into harmony. Furthermore, the sound at the throat tends to soothe one's whole being. If one remains aware of this sound for a reasonable period of time to the exclusion of other thoughts, the benefits are felt immediately.

When is ujjayi combined with other practices?

Swami Niranjanananda: Generally ujjayi pranayama is combined with various other practices. For example, often ujjayi breathing is used in the practice of nadi shodhana.

The practice of khechari mudra is combined with ujjayi pranayama as the throat does not become dry if the tongue is rolled up and placed at the root of the palate in khechari mudra. Yogis believe that with this combined practice of ujjayi and khechari mudra, the practice of ajapa japa can be perfected.

Gheranda Samhita (5:70–71) describes the practice of ujjayi with jalandhara bandha:

Naasaabhyaam vaayumaakrishya mukhamadhye cha dhaarayet; Hridgalaabhyaam samaakrishya vaayum vaktre cha dhaarayet.

Mukham prakshaalya samvandya kuryaajjaalandharam tatah; Aashakti kumbhakam kritvaa dhaarayedavirodhatah.

Inhaling external air through both the nostrils, suck the internal air through the heart and throat and hold it by means of kumbhaka. (70)

Then emptying the mouth, apply jalandhara bandha, and hold the breath to capacity in a manner which does not cause any obstruction. (71)

Although ujjayi is not often practised as a separate prana-yama, it can be used in this way.

When can ujjayi be incorporated into asana practice?

Swami Satyananda: Ujjayi can be incorporated into asana practice for specific therapeutic purposes, such as when practising makarasana for sciatica or spinal spondylitis, or shashankasana for menstrual tension, insomnia or emotional disturbance. It can also be incorporated into asana practice purely to increase the awareness and to stimulate sushumna.

Why is ujjayi used in subtle practices?

Swami Satyananda: Ujjayi is used in meditation practices, kriya yoga and prana vidya because it helps relax the physical body and the mind, and develops awareness of the subtle body and psychic sensitivity. Ujjayi promotes internalization of the senses and pratyahara.

When it is practised for relaxation and concentration of mind, it should be done after other pranayama techniques and before concentrating on a psychic symbol.

How does ujjayi prepare one for meditation?

Swami Satyananda: It is good to awaken *sushumna*, the middle passage of prana, for meditation. One should do this by pranayamas. In pranayama, there are a few methods which are necessary and useful for the practice of meditation. The best pranayama for this purpose is ujjayi. It is with the help of ujjayi pranayama that consciousness is brought to function in the system. After doing ujjayi about 50, 60, or 70 times, one is ready for meditation.

Why is ujjayi used in kriya yoga?

Swami Satyananda: Those spiritual seekers who want to break the bondage of matter over mind, and mind over spirit, will find out how difficult this is. To aid this process, ujjayi pranayama, psychic breathing, is used in most kriyas. There are many types of pranayama: nadi shodhana, bhastrika, kapalbhati, ujjayi, sheetali, sheetkari, bhramari, surya bheda, moorcha, etc. Out of all these, ujjayi pranayama is chosen for kriya yoga because it has been found that it is the easiest and safest. Bhastrika pranayama is faster and the results are quick but at the same time the side effects are uncertain. With ujjayi pranayama, the effect is slow but it is certain and safe.

When ujjayi is practised for fifteen minutes or half an hour, suddenly a feeling of slipping out of the body and being somewhere else arises. This is how yoga helps overcome physical, material, earthly problems and allows the seeker to fulfil the spiritual ambition which is cherished in the heart: to be one with the higher self, to break the bondage of maya, to overcome the mental limitations, to unite with the spirit. This is the mission of yoga in every country, and on every continent.

What is the kurma nadi and how does practising ujjayi influence it?

Swami Satyananda: It is said in the raja yoga of Sage Patanjali that there is a particular nadi in the shape of a turtle, or tortoise. It is situated in the vishuddhi region, not exactly in vishuddhi, but in the vishuddhi region – a little above anahata, a little below vishuddhi. If one concentrates on that particular nadi one attains control of the pranamaya kosha, or the energy waves of prana, that are exploding or manifesting in the body. Practise ujjayi pranayama and concentrate only within this area, neither up nor down. At that time it is said that the realization of the perception of the *kurma nadi*, the tortoise nerve, takes place.

Can ujjayi occur spontaneously?

Swami Satyananda: Although it is described as a specific practice, ujjayi often occurs spontaneously when concentration becomes deep and intense.

Why is ujjayi associated with pranic awakening?

Swami Niranjanananda: Awareness of the psychic breath is the first stage of unlocking the doors of the pranic body. The experience of the breath can be both gross and subtle. The gross experience is the physical process of inhalation and exhalation: one breathes in, one breathes out, one becomes aware of the breath in the nostrils, in the lungs, in the lower abdominal region, and in the chest. Manipulation of the physical breath through willpower, through concentration and the practices of pranayama, is the gross aspect of the breath.

The other aspect of the breath is psychic, the movement of inhalation and exhalation in the form of ujjayi pranayama. Awareness of the deep sound made in ujjayi pranayama during inhalation and exhalation is awareness of the psychic breath. Awareness of the psychic breath is not an unnatural or unconscious process, but involves the practice of awareness, concentration and actual physiological contraction of the throat muscles.

When ujjayi breathing is practised with khechari mudra and *nasikagra drishti*, nosetip gazing, instead of watching the normal flow of breath in the nostrils, one simply becomes aware of the breath passing in through the throat and the sound that it makes. How can this awareness open the door of the pranic body? It is very simple. When the breath is observed in the throat with total involvement of the senses, the mind relaxes, the activities of the brain slow down and new forms of experience shape themselves within the personality. When ujjayi is practised the actual physiological experience is one of tranquillity, relaxation and one-pointedness. This is the gross experience of ujjayi pranayama.

Then there is the psychic experience. With the practice of ujjayi the prana begins to move, the prana located in the chest begins to move. As ujjayi is practised using the prana moving within in the form of a stream of light particles, a sort of tickling or burning sensation is experienced in the

176

throat, in the upper thoracic region, chest and lungs. That is the first physiological experience that indicates possible pranic awakening. It is experienced as the concentration becomes deep and intense. In the practice of psychic breathing one tries to actually change the flow of prana.

MOORCHHA PRANAYAMA: THE FAINTING BREATH

What is moorchha pranayama?
Swami Satyananda: *Moorchha* means 'to faint' or 'to swoon'. Through this pranayama the experience of conscious unconsciousness is meant to arise, but it must be learned under expert guidance.

Why does the sensation of fainting occur when practising moorchha pranayama?
Swami Satyananda: The sensation of fainting occurs for two reasons. One is that continued retention lowers the oxygen concentration in the blood reaching the brain (hypoxia). Secondly, by compressing the great vessels in the neck, *jalandhara bandha*, the chin lock, influences the pressure receptors in their walls and the heart rate and blood pressure are adjusted by the reflex response. In *Hatha Yoga Pradipika* (2:69) it is said:

> *Poorantake gaadhataram badhva jaalandharam shanaih;*
> *Rechayenmoorchchanaakhyeyam manomoorchchaa sukhapradaa.*

> At the end of inhalation gradually become fixed on jalandhara bandha, then exhale slowly. This is called the fainting or swooning pranayama as it makes the mind inactive and thus confers pleasure.

The word moorchha implies insensibility of mind, meaning the conscious mind. This pranayama clears the mind of unnecessary thoughts and reduces awareness of the senses and external world, producing a psychic state of introversion. Therefore, it is an excellent preparation for meditation and enhances concentration, practices. It helps reduce anxiety and mental tension, inducing relaxation and inner awareness.

When is a practitioner ready to practise moorchha pranayama?

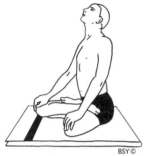
Moorchha Pranayama

Swami Satyananda: Moorchha pranayama is only to be done by advanced practitioners who have purified their bodies and who have a good capacity to retain the breath. With practice, the number of rounds can be increased and gradually extended from five minutes up to ten minutes. However, if there is any feeling of lightheadedness, the practice must be stopped.

What precautions should be observed when practising moorchha pranayama?

Swami Niranjanananda: As the technique induces the sensation of swooning or light-headedness, it should only be practised under the guidance of a competent teacher. In a favourable environment, with complete self-purification, proper diet, etc., it is not difficult to retain the breath for longer durations. However, without the necessary preparations, extended breath retention should not be practised, as it can be harmful.

This technique should not be practised by those suffering from heart disease, high blood pressure, epilepsy, brain disorders or atherosclerosis of the carotid or basilar arteries.

Practitioners are cautioned against excessive practising of moorchha pranayama as fainting can occur. The purpose is to disassociate the consciousness from the physical world and the complexities of the mind, and to be lifted above awareness of the physical body. Such a state is swooning or semi-fainting, not complete unconsciousness. The practice should be discontinued if a strong fainting sensation is felt.

178

What are the effects of moorchha pranayama?

Swami Niranjanananda: *Moorchha* means becoming unconscious. The practitioner of this pranayama becomes unconscious of the material world, and another state of consciousness is attained. Attachment to the manifest world and body starts to fade and the mind becomes peaceful. This is described in *Gheranda Samhita* (5:85):

> *Sukhena kumbhakam kritvaa manashcha bhruvorantaram;*
> *Santyajya vishayaansarvaanmanomoorchchhaa sukhapradaa;*
> *Aatmani manaso yogaadaanando jaayate dhruvam.*

> Perform breath retention comfortably. Take the mind away from material things and focus it on the eyebrow centre, merging it with the atman. By perfecting moorchha kumbhaka, bliss is certainly attained.

Breath retention reduces the supply of oxygen to the brain. This is experienced particularly when the breath is held for longer durations. The brain becomes less alert and a sensation of swooning starts to dawn. In moorchha pranayama breath retention is of special significance and while practising this pranayama, the longer the breath retention, the better the results. Breath retention's direct effect on the mind via the pranic body is the automatic stopping of thoughts.

Moorchha pranayama is a powerful practice. Sage Gheranda says that a person who masters this practice experiences psychic bliss. As the duration of internal breath retention increases, the bliss also increases.

This practice draws the mind inwards and enables a psychic state to be experienced. It cuts out the distractions of the external world, inhibits identification with the physical body and brings about mental tranquillity. An experience of lightness arises with this practice. Tension, anxiety, anger and neuroses are alleviated, and there is a letting go of attachment to sensory experiences. A state of void is induced spontaneously. Therefore, moorchha pranayama is an excellent preparation for meditation.

179

CHANDRA BHEDA PRANAYAMA:
THE MOON PIERCING BREATH

What is chandra bheda pranayama?

Swami Niranjanananda: *Chandra* means 'moon' and indicates ida nadi. *Bhedan* means 'to pierce'. This pranayama pierces ida nadi and fills it with shakti by breathing in through the left nostril only and out through the right nostril only. In this way there is a predominant stimulation of the parasympathetic nervous system and right brain hemisphere. This practice should only be done under expert guidance, as the awakened forces of manas shakti are not controlled easily. Generally, this technique is not publicized. Chandra bheda pranayama is described in the *Yoga Chudamani Upanishad* (v. 95–96):

> *Baddhapadmaasano yogee pranam chandrena poorayet;*
> *Dhaarayedvaa yathaashaktyaa bhooyah sooryena rechayet.*

> *Amritodadhisandhisankaasham goksheeradhavalopamam;*
> *Dhyaatvaa chandramasam bimbam praanaayaame sukhee bhavet.*

(Sitting) in baddha padmasana, the yogi should inhale the breath through the left nostril, retain it for as long as possible, and exhale again through the right nostril. (95)

At the time of pranayama one should meditate on the luminous disc of the moon, which is like the ocean of nectar and white like the milk of cows. (96)

Why is surya bheda pranayama more widely known than chandra bheda pranayama?

Swami Satyananda: *Surya bheda pranayama* activates the pingala nadi, which is responsible for the physical actions, and which carries the flow of the life force. If this pranayama is practised in the reverse manner, inhaling though the left nostril and exhaling through the right, it activates ida nadi, the energy of the mind, as represented by the moon, and is known as *chandra bheda pranayama*.

In *Hatha Yoga Pradipika*, nothing is written about this pranayama because if ida is awakened the mind can introvert completely and the body will become lethargic. Yoga does not want any acceleration in the mental activity of a yogi, as the purpose of yoga is to calm down the turbulent tendencies of the mind. Consequently this practice is unknown. It is quite safe to activate pingala nadi through surya bheda pranayama, but it can be dangerous to activate ida through chandra bheda unless the guru has specifically advised it.

BHRAMARI: THE HUMMING BEE BREATH

What is bhramari pranayama?

Swami Satyananda: Bhramari, 'the humming bee' pranayama, is so called because the sound made during respiration imitates that of a black bee. *Hatha Yoga Pradipika* (2:68) speaks highly of bhramari:

Vegaadghosham poorakam bhringanaadam bhringeenaadam rechakam mandamandam;
Yogeendraanaamevamabhyaasayogaachchitte jaataa kaachidaanandaleelaa.

Breathe in quickly, making a reverberating sound like the male black bee, and exhale slowly while softly making the sound of the female black bee. By this yogic practice one becomes lord of the yogis and the mind is absorbed in bliss.

What are the benefits of practising bhramari?

Swami Niranjanananda: Bhramari relieves stress and cerebral tension, alleviating anger, anxiety and insomnia, and reducing blood pressure. It speeds up the healing capacity of the body and may be practised after operations. It strengthens and improves the voice and eliminates throat ailments. Bhramari induces a meditative state by harmonizing the mind and directing the awareness inward. It leads to spontaneous meditative experience, inner perception, bliss and ultimately to mastery of samadhi.

Why is the practice of bhramari ideal for busy people?

Swami Niranjanananda: Bhramari pranayama has a deeply soothing effect on the nerves, especially for those people who are physically and mentally in a rush. It has been found that bhramari stimulates alpha brainwaves. When one is in a rush, there are certain simple breathing practices that can be performed, and bhramari pranayama is one of them. The sound produced in bhramari is very soothing and the practice reduces mental tension, anxiety and anger.

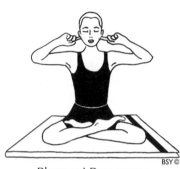

Bhramari Pranayama

What time of day is best for practising bhramari?

Swami Satyananda: Bhramari helps to awaken psychic sensitivity and awareness of subtle vibrations; this is why it is better to practise in the early hours of the morning or late at night when there are few external sounds. However, bhramari may be practised at any time to relieve mental tension, provided the surroundings are peaceful.

How much time should one spend practising bhramari?

Swami Niranjanananda: In the beginning, five to ten rounds are sufficient. As experience is gained, one can slowly increase to ten to fifteen minutes. In cases of extreme mental tension or anxiety, or when being used to assist the healing process, practise for up to thirty minutes. For spiritual purposes bhramari may be continued for longer periods.

What precautions should be observed when practising bhramari?

Swami Niranjanananda: Bhramari should not be performed while lying down. People suffering from severe ear infections should not practise this pranayama until the infection has cleared up. Those with heart disease must practise without breath retention.

Where should the awareness be focused while practising bhramari?

Swami Satyananda: During bhramari pranayama, concentrate on the source of the sound in the brain and the effect of the gentle humming vibrations.

Is bhramari a pranayama or a practice of nada yoga?

Swami Satyananda: Bhramari is both a pranayama and a practice of nada yoga. It is practised in a sitting position. In the scriptures, the heart centre is termed 'the centre of unstruck sound', and also, 'the cave of the bees'. In bhramari pranayama the humming sound of the bees is produced and traced towards its source. This produces deep mental and emotional relaxation, making it extremely useful for those with cardiac disorders and other diseases characterized by a high level of mental tension, such as epilepsy and asthma.

However, it must be learned correctly, because the whole process is subtle. It is a process of inner absorption into the humming sound, which is produced with gentle exhalation. The practice must take place effortlessly, without any strain to prolong the vibration unduly, or to make it loud. It should be spontaneous and it can be very soft. It is essentially an internal sound, and when the ears are blocked with the fingers, the practitioner continues to follow the inner vibration and discover the source.

8

Vitalizing Pranayamas

ABOUT VITALIZING PRANAYAMAS

What are the characteristics of the vitalizing pranayamas?
Swami Niranjanananda: All pranayamas are vitalizing in the sense that they enhance the pranic system. However, the techniques which are categorized as vitalizing do so in a dynamic way, arousing body and mind, creating alertness and heat at both the physical and subtle levels. The tranquillizing techniques are cooling and soothing, while the vitalizing techniques produce the opposite effect. The vitalizing pranayamas can be used to increase the energy or to move out of introspective or dull states of mind.

When is a student ready to learn vitalizing pranayamas?
Swami Niranjanananda: Vitalizing pranayamas are regarded as more advanced techniques which are introduced after mastering yogic breathing and practising nadi shodhana for some time. They should not be practised in hot weather or before sleep.

SWANA PRANAYAMA: THE PANTING BREATH

What is swana pranayama?
Swami Niranjanananda: *Swana* means 'panting'. It is actually a simple form of agnisara kriya. In swana pranayama,

184

abdominal movement is combined with oral respiration. The word 'agnisara' is very meaningful in this context. *Agni* means 'fire', *sara* means 'movement'. This practice is the movement of the fire element which is centralized in the visceral area from where the heat mechanism is stimulated. Agnisara kriya uses bahir kumbhaka at the time of moving the abdomen, whereas swana pranayama involves rapid respiration using the same abdominal movement. This is a different action from normal abdominal breathing, which uses the diaphragm. With swana pranayama, the abdominal muscles themselves are used.

What are the benefits of swana pranayama?

Swami Niranjanananda: Swana pranayama improves digestion, tones the visceral organs, muscles, nerves and blood vessels. Fatty tissue on the abdomen is reduced and the lungs are emptied of stale air. It helps relieve flatulence, constipation, poor digestion and loss of appetite.

Swana pranayama is a useful preparation for bhastrika and kapalbhati pranayamas.

When should swana pranayama be practised or not be practised?

Swami Niranjanananda: Swana pranayama should be done on an empty stomach or at least four hours after eating. It should not be attempted by people suffering from stomach or intestinal ulcers, hernia, heart disease, high blood pressure, overactive thyroid gland or chronic diarrhoea.

BHASTRIKA PRANAYAMA: THE BELLOWS BREATH

What is bhastrika pranayama?

Swami Satyananda: *Bhastra* are the bellows used to fan a fire. Thus the practice can be called 'the bellows pranayama'. This practice is so called because air is drawn forcefully and quickly in and out of the lungs as through the bellows of a village blacksmith. The blacksmith increases the flow of air into a fire in order to produce more heat for his work. Bhastrika pranayama can be said to do the same thing: it increases the flow of air into the body, producing inner heat, both gross and subtle. The inner fire of the mind-body is stoked. This heat burns up impurities, whether physical impurities such as toxins, pranic blockages, or mental neuroses. The Sanskrit word *tapas* means 'to burn one's impurities'. Bhastrika pranayama is one method, a most direct method of self-purification through tapas. Bhastrika is described in *Gheranda Samhita* (5:76–78):

Bhastrikaa lohakaaraanaam yathaakramena sambhramet;
Tathaa vaayum cha naasaabhyaamubhaabhyaam chaalayechchhanaih.

Evam vinshativaaram cha kritvaa kuryaachcha kumbhakam;
Tadante chaalayedvaayum poorvoktam cha yathaavidhi.

Trivaaram saadhayedenam bhastrikaakumbhakam sudheeh;
Na cha rogo na cha klesha aarogyam cha dine dine.

Breathe in and out forcefully through both nostrils, filling and emptying the abdomen like the bellows of a blacksmith. (76)

Repeat this 20 times then hold the breath. The learned ones have named it bhastrika kumbhaka. It should be repeated thus thrice. By practising it, no disease or disorder takes place and a disease-free state is increased day by day. (77–78)

How should one prepare for practising bhastrika?

Swami Niranjanananda: When practising bhastrika both nostrils must be clear and flowing freely. Mucus blockages can be removed by neti. If the swara is greatly imbalanced, then one of the balancing methods may be used prior to the practice.

Beginners should be familiar with abdominal (diaphragmatic) breathing before starting. Proficiency in antar and bahir kumbhaka, as well as jalandhara, uddiyana and moola bandhas are necessary before introducing the later stages of practice. Control of the nostrils is through nasagra mudra; the thumb controlling the right nostril, the ring finger controlling the left.

What are the different levels of practising bhastrika?

Swami Niranjanananda: Bhastrika is graded into four techniques. Techniques 1 and 2 are at beginner's level as they establish the basic method of practice. Technique 3, the intermediate level, increases the number of breaths in each round, introduces internal kumbhaka, and moola and jalandhara bandhas. Technique 4, the advanced level, introduces external kumbhaka and maha bandha, and increases the number of rounds further.

The practitioner should proceed slowly and be sensitive to his own capacity. Each technique should be practised until it has been consolidated before proceeding to the next. Bhastrika may be practised at three degrees of intensity: slow, medium and fast, depending on the capacity of the practitioner.

What are the guidelines for practising bhastrika as a sadhana?

Swami Satyananda: Before commencing bhastrika, those who have never practised pranayama before must first take up other preliminary practices. Nadi shodhana should be practised as the preliminary pranayama, gradually increasing the ratios and duration of retention. Nadi shodhana can be continued during any season and, excluding retention, it may be done by anyone. There are specific requirements for bhastrika pranayama, and one should not perform it without the guru's instructions.

What precautions should be observed in relation to bhastrika?

Swami Niranjanananda: Bhastrika is a dynamic practice requiring a large expenditure of physical energy, and must

187

be practised in a relaxed manner. Beginners who are not used to using the abdominal muscles correctly are advised to take a few normal breaths and a short rest after each round. A feeling of faintness, excessive perspiration or a nauseous sensation indicates that the practice is being performed incorrectly. Avoid violent respiration, as the speed of the breath should be controlled. Avoid facial contortions and excessive shaking of the body. If any of these symptoms are experienced, the advice of a yoga teacher should be sought. A slow, conscientious approach is recommended.

Bhastrika should not be practised by people who suffer from high blood pressure, heart disease, hernia, gastric ulcer, stroke, epilepsy, retinal problems, glaucoma or vertigo. Those suffering from lung diseases such as asthma and chronic bronchitis, those recovering from tuberculosis, or in the first trimester of pregnancy are recommended to practise only under expert guidance.

Bhastrika purifies the blood. However, if the stages are rushed, all the impurities will be ejected from the body in a rush, which may exacerbate conditions caused by detoxification. A slow, conscientious approach to this practice is absolutely imperative. Bhastrika is full, rapid breathing. Hypoventilation can occur if the air is not fully expelled from the lungs on each exhalation. This is another indication that the technique is not being performed correctly.

What are the overall benefits of bhastrika?

Swami Satyananda: Generally, it can be said that bhastrika supercharges the entire physical-pranic-mental body. One's whole being becomes sensitive and one becomes more receptive to higher and more subtle vibrations. Such is the utility of bhastrika pranayama.

Physically, bhastrika speeds up the blood circulation, allowing the organs, muscles, nerves, etc., of the body to function more efficiently. It also improves digestion by giving a vigorous massage to the digestive organs, leading to better all-round health. It removes physical impurities by increasing the metabolic rate and increasing blood circulation. Bhastrika is therefore a first rate technique for purifying the blood, improving skin complexion and removing eruptions such as boils and pimples.

At the energetic level, bhastrika increases the flow of prana throughout the whole pranic body, helping to induce good health and remove disease at more subtle levels. The pranic body is recharged. Pranic movement, particularly in the coccygeal, navel, thoracic and brain centres, is accelerated by the practice of bhastrika, increasing physical vitality and bestowing clarity of mind. Bhastrika, therefore, makes the mind one-pointed, preparing the body-mind for meditation. The tremendous heat generated by the practice clears sushumna nadi and prepares it for the ascent of kundalini.

Why is bhastrika a purifying practice?

Swami Satyananda: Bhastrika is ideal for purifying the blood and improving a bad complexion. However, this purification should be slow. If too much bhastrika is done, then all the impurities in the blood will be ejected from the body in a mighty torrent. This may result in massive boils or other skin eruptions in the initial stages of practice. One should proceed steadily but surely. Let the impurities be removed slowly. In this manner painful boils or skin eruptions are less likely.

What are the physiological effects of bhastrika?

Swami Satyananda: The most important physiological effect of bhastrika is on the brain and heart. Bhastrika stimulates the circulation of cerebral fluid and increases the compression and decompression on the brain, creating a rhythmic massage. The rhythmic pumping of the diaphragm and lungs stimulates the heart and blood circulation. Accelerated blood circulation and rate of gaseous exchange in each cell produces heat and 'washes out' waste gases. Hyperventilation begins to occur and excites the sympathetic nerves in the respiratory centre, but because there is an increased release

189

of carbon dioxide, the centre is subsequently relaxed and hyperventilation does not take place. If exhalation were to become less than inhalation, there would be hyperventilation. Therefore, in bhastrika inhalation and exhalation must remain equal.

The rapid and rhythmic movement of the diaphragm stimulates the visceral organs creating a massaging effect throughout the internal system. Bhastrika and kapalbhati are the most dynamic and vitalizing pranayama techniques. Bhastrika heats the nasal passages and sinuses, clearing away excess mucus and building up resistance to colds and all respiratory disorders, therefore it is useful in the yogic management of chronic sinusitis, pleurisy, asthma and bronchitis. Bhastrika improves digestion and stimulates a sluggish system. It increases the appetite, accelerates the metabolic rate and strengthens the nervous system. Bhastrika also helps in cases of tuberculosis, constipation, sciatica, spondylitis, arthritis, rheumatic problems, cancer and physical and mental tension.

What is the effect of bhastrika on the lungs and the normal breathing pattern?

Swami Satyananda: Most people do not breathe properly – the breathing tends to be shallow. The lungs are not fully used and exercised, and the small air sacs (alveoli) in the lower lobes of the lungs tend to stay permanently closed. Mucus builds up and acts as fertile soil for the growth of germs and disease. When the alveoli remain permanently closed the blood is not fully oxygenated. Those parts of the lungs that are open allow oxygen-carbon dioxide exchange, while the closed or blocked parts don't. This results in 'mismatching', a condition where one part of the lungs gives more transfer than other parts. The overall effect is decreased oxygen content in the blood. That is, instead of an ideal one hundred percent oxygenation there may only be seventy percent. This results in decreased oxygenation of the body tissues and general weakness and bad health.

Bhastrika directly opens up closed alveoli. Germs, mucus and possibly stagnant air are eliminated from the lungs. All the alveoli, the little air sacs, are cleaned and rejuvenated from top to bottom, which leads to an increased transfer of oxygen through the cell membranes and allows better removal of waste carbon dioxide from the body. This results in improved overall health and increased vitality. Bhastrika purifies the lungs, making it a useful technique for combating ailments such as asthma, tuberculosis, pleurisy and bronchitis.

Most people do not use their abdomen when they breathe. Bhastrika is a means of retraining the nerve reflexes of the body so that there is increased use of the abdominal muscles during normal respiration throughout the day. Deeper breathing means that the body induces abundant amounts of oxygen with the minimum number of breaths. This means that the body cells obtain adequate nutrition in the form of oxygen with minimum energy expenditure.

What are the effects of bhastrika on the body and mind?

Swami Niranjanananda: When bhastrika is practised systematically and conscientiously, the benefits are innumerable. Due to the rapid exchange of air in the lungs, there is an increase in the exchange of oxygen and carbon dioxide into and out of the bloodstream. This stimulates the metabolic rate throughout the body down to the cellular level, producing heat and flushing out wastes and toxins. If one is caught in the cold without sufficient warm clothing, bhastrika can be practised to warm the body quickly.

Bhastrika is a process of hyperventilation, leading to respiratory alkalosis, which has a soothing effect on the respiratory centre. It reduces the level of carbon dioxide in the blood; hence a better kumbhaka can be performed after the practice. The rapid and rhythmic movement of the diaphragm also massages and stimulates the visceral organs, toning the digestive system and improving its blood circulation. The massage also strengthens the muscles of the intestines and other organs in the abdominal cavity, providing the organs adequate support from the front, so that they do not cause a stretch on the lumbar spine, which is often the cause of lower back pain. It is a useful practice for women during labour, if they have had proper preparation.

Bhastrika helps balance the *doshas* or humours: *kapha*, phlegm; *pitta*, bile; and *vata*, wind. It helps to alleviate inflammation in the throat, accumulation of phlegm and sinusitis, and builds up resistance to coughs, colds and excess mucus. It also balances and strengthens the nervous system, inducing peace, tranquillity and one-pointedness of mind. Hysteria, psychosis and chronic depression respond well to bhastrika.

The practice of bhastrika increases vitality and lowers levels of stress and anxiety by raising the energy and harmonizing the pranas. It increases the generation of samana vayu, which replenishes the pranic store and stimulates the whole pranic system. While practising, all the pranas in the body begin to vibrate, but at the end of the practice the mind is completely stilled. In fact, the meditative state can be reached effortlessly through the practice of bhastrika. The yogic texts state that bhastrika enables prana to break through the three knots in the sushumna passage, making way for the kundalini shakti to flow upwards freely.

What is the effect of bhastrika on the doshas?

Swami Niranjanananda: This practice burns up toxins and removes diseases of the doshas or humours: *kapha*, phlegm, *pitta*, bile and *vata*, wind. It alleviates inflammation in the throat and any accumulated phlegm. It is recommended for asthmatics and those suffering from other lung disorders.

What is the role of the diaphragm in bhastrika?

Swami Niranjanananda: In bhastrika the action of the diaphragm and the abdominal muscles are exactly like bellows. The ribcage muscles play only a minimal role. The diaphragm is used to create equal force on inhalation (relaxing on exhalation) and the abdominal muscles are

192

used to create force on exhalation (relaxing on inhalation). Both create a pull-push action. Concentration just below the sternum will help. Only the abdomen moves in and out during the practice. There should be no other movement in the body; it should be like a statue, regardless of the velocity bhastrika attains.

One may close the eyes during the practice. If the eyes are kept open, they should be fixed on a point. In either case, there should be total steadiness throughout the practice. When attempting bhastrika for the first time, a loss in power and coordination of the diaphragm and abdominal muscles may be felt after a few rounds. This occurs due to insufficient toning and control of these muscles. Further preparation and consolidation of this technique would be necessary before proceeding. One should be able to perform the basic method with ease before proceeding to the other techniques.

If bhastrika is practised during the hot season, do five to ten rounds of sheetali or sheetkari pranayama afterwards to cool the body.

What are the effects of bhastrika on the nervous and pranic systems?

Swami Niranjanananda: Bhastrika activates the brain and induces clarity of thought and concentration. Vitality is increased and the pranas are harmonized, reducing stress and anxiety levels. Pranic blockages are cleared, causing sushumna nadi to flow, which leads to deep states of meditation and spiritual awakening. Bhastrika balances and strengthens the nervous system, inducing peace, tranquillity and one-pointedness of mind in preparation for meditation.

How can bhastrika be used as a pathway to meditation?

Swami Satyananda: Concentration during bhastrika must be on counting the breaths, up to 100, 200, 300, 400, or more. Kumbhaka is then held with uddiyana, jalandhara and moola bandhas and concentration respectively on mooladhara, manipura and vishuddhi chakras, followed by correct release of the bandhas. In this way, another round should be practised. If one can hold the awareness, the quality and depth of *dharana*, concentration, will improve. In fact, *dhyana*, meditation, results from deep concentration in bhastrika.

What are the physical, pranic and psychic benefits of bhastrika?

Swami Sivananda: Bhastrika relieves inflammation of the throat, increases gastric fire, destroys phlegm, removes diseases of the nose and chest including asthma and consumption, and ensures a good appetite. It gives warmth to the body. In a cool region, practise this pranayama to protect the body from cold – it will quickly generate sufficient warmth in the body.

Bhastrika is the most beneficial of all kumbhakas. It purifies the nadis and enables the prana to break through the three *granthis* or knots in sushumna, namely brahma granthi, vishnu granthi and rudra granthi. It destroys phlegm which is the bolt or obstacle to the door at the mouth of sushumna nadi, and enables one to know the kundalini. The practitioner of bhastrika will never suffer from any disease. He will always be healthy.

What is the effect of bhastrika on the granthis?

Swami Satyananda: Within sushumna there are three granthis or psychic/pranic knots which prevent the passage of kundalini shakti. One is found in mooladhara chakra. It is called *brahma granthi* and it ties the awareness to sensual perception and the physical world. Another is in anahata chakra and it causes the desire for emotional security, expression and fulfilment. It is called *vishnu granthi*. The third granthi is located in ajna chakra and is associated with attachment to siddhis, psychic phenomena and experiences. It is called *rudra granthi*. The shakti produced by bhastrika is said to break these granthis so that kundalini can move on unobstructed. *Hatha Yoga Pradipika* (2:66–67), describes the process:

Kundalee bodhakam kshipram pavanam sukhadam hitam;
Brahmanaadeemukhe samsthakaphaadyargalanaashanam.

Samyaggaatrasamudbhootagranthitrayavibhedakam;
Visheshenaiva kartavyam bhastraakhyam kumbhakamtvidam.

This (bhastrika) quickly arouses kundalini. It is pleasant and beneficial, and removes obstruction due to excess mucus accumulated at the entrance to brahma nadi. (66)

This kumbhaka called bhastrika enables the three granthis to be broken. Thus it is the duty of the yogi to practise bhastrika. (67)

Through the practice of bhastrika, the *indriyas* – the *jnanendriyas*, sensory organs, and the *karmendriyas*, motor organs – become less influential in motivating one's behaviour, and the need for sensual enjoyment decreases. The nervous system becomes stronger, the emotions are harmonized and deeper inner satisfaction results. This occurs when brahma and vishnu granthis begin to loosen. When psychic experiences begin, bhastrika helps one to remain a silent uninvolved witness who is not attached to any of these experiences. As rudra granthi starts to release, this attitude of *sakshi*, the witness, develops.

It is not easy to loosen the granthis because there are many physical, emotional and mental barriers. For the average person it is almost impossible to control sensual desires and to live without emotional security and fulfilment. As for psychic experiences, those who have them often end up in a mental hospital because they have no guru to guide them through their spiritual awakening.

Therefore, although bhastrika helps loosen the granthis which obstruct kundalini's ascent, it is not enough just to practise bhastrika for hours together; a guru's guidance is necessary.

What are the spiritual effects of bhastrika?

Swami Satyananda: The number one practice in the awakening of kundalini is bhastrika. Bhastrika pranayama powerfully influences the nervous system and brain. By regular practice it can completely alter habitual neuronal firing patterns in the brain, particularly in the regions of the recticular activating system and hypothalamus. It thereby modifies the basic and deep-rooted emotional responses of the personality, of which fear of death is primal. This powerful effect is mentioned in *Hatha Yoga Pradipika* (3:122):

> *Kundaleem chaalayitvaa tu bhastraam kuryaardvisheshatah;*
> *Evamabhyasato nityam yamino yamabheeh kutah.*

> Bhastrika pranayama with kumbhaka should specifically be practised to activate kundalini. From where will the fear of death arise for a self-restrained practitioner who practises daily with regularity?

However, the process of emergence of a yogic personality is an evolutionary transformation which is gradual and painstaking. It is said that a yogi transcends the fear of death altogether, and it becomes a challenge for death to overtake him.

KAPALBHATI PRANAYAMA:
FRONTAL BRAIN CLEANSING TECHNIQUE

What is kapalbhati?

Swami Satyananda: The last of the six shatkarmas in *Hatha Yoga Pradipika* and *Gheranda Samhita* is kapalbhati. *Kapala* means the 'cranium' or 'forehead'. *Bhati* is 'light' or 'splendour', but it also means 'perception and knowledge'. Kapalbhati is a pranayama technique which invigorates the entire brain and awakens the dormant centres which are responsible for subtle perception. In English it is called the 'frontal brain cleansing' technique. *Hatha Yoga Pradipika* (2:35) describes the way of breathing as being like a bellows:

Bhastraavallohakaarasya rechapoorau sasambhramau;
Kapaalabhaatirvikhyaa kaphadoshavishoshanee.

Perform exhalation and inhalation rapidly like the
bellows (of a blacksmith). This is called kapalbhati; it
destroys all mucous disorders.

Kapalbhati is a similar practice to bhastrika pranayama
except that exhalation is emphasized and inhalation is the
result of forcing the air out. In normal breathing, inhalation
is active and exhalation is passive. Kapalbhati reverses that
process so that exhalation becomes active and inhalation
passive. This is like the pumping action of the blacksmith's
bellows; when the bellows are closed the air is pushed out,
and when they are opened the air is sucked in due to the
vacuum effect that is created. Similarly, when one inhales in
kapalbhati, it should be a reaction to the forced exhalation.

**What is the difference between practising kapalbhati as a
shatkarma and as a pranayama?**
Swami Niranjanananda: When it is performed as a shatkarma,
kapalbhati clears excess mucus from the nasal passages and
should be practised before pranayama.

**Why is kapalbhati classified as a shatkarma when it is a
pranayama technique?**
Swami Satyananda: Kapalbhati is a shatkarma, but it is also a
pranayama. Whereas other pranayamas require a somewhat
purified system, kapalbhati does not, as it purifies; so it
comes under the shatkarmas.

**Why is kapalbhati the sixth shatkarma in *Gheranda
Samhita*?**
Swami Niranjanananda: In *Gheranda Samhita* the first five
groups of shatkarmas: dhauti, basti, neti, nauli and trataka,
aim to cleanse or purify the organs of the body, and to
achieve mental concentration and stability. The sixth
shatkarma, kapalbhati, is for the purification of pranamaya

kosha. It has also been known as bhalbhati, but kapalbhati is now a more common name. *Kapala* means 'skull', *bhal* means 'forehead', *bhati* means 'light'. In *Gheranda Samhita* (1:55) three types of kapalbhati are named:

Vaatakramena vyutkramena sheetkramena visheshatah;
Bhaalabhaatim tridhaa kuryaatkaphadosham nivaarayet.

Vatakrama, vyutkrama and sheetkrama are the three types of bhalbhati. Practising them eliminates phlegm and mucus from the body.

Sage Gheranda discusses three practices which are all variations of bhalbhati or kapalbhati. The first, *vatakrama*, uses air. The second and third, *vyutkrama* and *sheetkrama* use water in a manner similar to jala neti.

What is the difference between kapalbhati and bhastrika?
Swami Niranjanananda: Although kapalbhati is similar to bhastrika, there are important differences. In bhastrika the breathing rate increases with practice while in kapalbhati the speed becomes slower and slower. As one progresses in bhastrika, the breath gets faster and shorter; whereas in kapalbhati the breath is faster in the beginning, but with practice becomes slower and longer.

Bhastrika uses equal force in both inhalation and exhalation, expanding and contracting the thoracic area above and below its resting or basal volume. Kapalbhati, however, uses forced exhalation only, reducing the thoracic volume in exhalation, while inhalation remains a restful process from extreme exhalation to the basal volume. In normal breathing inhalation is active and exhalation passive. Kapalbhati reverses this procedure, making exhalation a forced, active process, while inhalation remains the same restful process.

Kapalbhati further reverses the natural process by compressing the lungs below basal resting volume, whereas normal breathing expands and contracts the lungs, using an active process on inhalation and a passive process on exhalation. The brain centres which control normal breathing function are trained to become more versatile through the practice of these techniques.

What are the different kapalbhati techniques within the hatha yoga tradition?

Swami Niranjanananda: *Gheranda Samhita* describes three types of kapalbhati. One of them resembles the practice given in *Hatha Yoga Pradipika*. Both these techniques use air, Sage Gheranda's version being named *vatakrama kapalbhati*. However, the technique is slightly different.

The major difference between the method of kapalbhati in the two traditions is that in the *Hatha Yoga Pradipika* of Yogi Swatmarama, there is no mention of breathing through alternate nostrils. It can be assumed that this is a preparation for Yogi Swatmarama's version of bhastrika pranayama. As with other shatkarmas, Yogi Swatmarama seems to deal with the shatkarmas at a more introductory level than Sage Gheranda.

Hatharatnavali (1:54–55) describes kapalbhati performed both with and without alternating the nostrils:

Atha kapaalabhaatih:
Bhastrivallauhakaaraanaam rechapoorasusambhramau;
Kapaalabhraantirvikhyaataa sarvarogavishoshanee.

Kapaalam bhraamayetsavyamapasavyam tu vegatah;
Rechapoorvakamuktena kapaalabhraantiruchyate.

Now kapalabhati:
Rapid performance of inhalation and exhalation like the bellows of the blacksmith is kapalbhati, well known as the destroyer of all diseases. (54)

Fast rotation of breathing from left to right and right to left, and exhalation and inhalation is called kapalbhati. (55)

What is involved in the practice of vatakrama kapalbhati?

Swami Niranjanananda: Vatakrama kapalbhati is described in *Gheranda Samhita* as one of the cleansing practices. As it uses air to clean the nasal area, it is also considered to be a type of pranayama. After inhaling, the air is expelled quickly, just as a blacksmith firing a furnace expels air from his bellows. On inhalation, air is allowed to enter the body passively, at a normal speed. In *Gheranda Samhita* (1:56–57) instructions are given:

Idayaa poorayedvaayum rechayetpingalayaa punah;
Pingalayaa poorayitvaa punashchandrena rechayet.

Poorakam rechakam kritvaa vegena na tu dhaarayet;
Evamabhyaasa yogena kapha dosham nivaarayet.

The breath is to be inhaled through ida nadi (the left nostril) and exhaled through pingala nadi (the right nostril). Then the breath is inhaled through surya nadi (the right nostril) and exhaled through chandra nadi (the left nostril). (56)

Inhalation and exhalation should be fast; do not hold it. This technique removes kapha dosha. (57)

Vatakrama kapalbhati is a difficult practice, as along with the forced exhalation, energy is focused through only one nostril at a time. Also, in this practice, awareness is taken to the forehead on exhalation, rather than to the abdomen as is usually the case in this type of vitalizing pranayama.

How does vatakrama kapalbhati benefit the respiratory system?

Swami Niranjanananda: With the practice of vatakrama kapalbhati fresh air reaches the lower peripheries of the lungs, while stale air is expelled. During this practice the respiratory system is activated, and the exchange of oxygen and carbon dioxide is increased. This practice benefits people suffering from respiratory ailments, including chronic bronchitis and tuberculosis.

People suffering from severe asthma and chronic lung disease often develop a habit of using the accessory muscles of respiration to breathe forcibly, and also tend to exhale with increased muscular force, making the muscles tired and causing fatigue. Such people should practise kapalbhati, but not while having an asthma attack.

What effect does vatakrama kapalbhati have on the brain?

Swami Niranjanananda: In the normal breathing process, the muscles of respiration – the diaphragm and intercostal muscles – actively contract during inhalation. During exhalation they generally relax passively: one has to make an effort to breathe in, whereas no effort is required for exhalation. Vatakrama kapalbhati reverses this natural process – the exhalation requires effort and is active, while the inhalation is natural or passive. This causes different neuronal pathways within the brain to fire and thus helps to awaken dormant brain centres.

Vatakrama kapalbhati increases cardiac output. With the increased blood flow, the frontal brain is purified and becomes more active. At the subtle level, prana shakti flows more strongly in this region of the brain. As well as bringing about improvement in the respiratory system and abdomen, vatakrama kapalbhati is one of the best practices for purification of this frontal part of the brain. It is a powerful technique for making the mind peaceful and aware.

How does vatakrama kapalbhati benefit the abdominal region?

Swami Niranjanananda: Vatakrama kapalbhati activates the muscles involved in exhalation, mainly the abdominal muscles, thus increasing the blood flow to them. At the same time, the digestive organs are activated, massaged and strengthened.

How many rounds of kapalbhati can be safely practised?

Swami Satyananda: In kapalbhati a greater number of respirations can be taken than in bhastrika pranayama, as hyperventilation does not occur. Up to two hundred breaths can be taken after months of practice, unless advised otherwise by one's guru.

If dizziness is experienced while practising, it means the breathing is too forceful. If this occurs, the practice should be stopped and recommenced after a few minutes of quiet sitting. When it is resumed, it should be done with more awareness and less force. There should not be a feeling of breathlessness before completing the round.

Where should the awareness be held during kapalbhati?

Swami Niranjanananda: The mind should be fixed at chidakasha, the dark empty space inside the forehead. With the eyes closed, one looks into this space. The lungs should move like a bellows. One feels pranic vibrations in chidakasha, and also feels that the frontal part of the brain is being purified.

When should kapalbhati be practised and for how long?

Swami Niranjanananda: Kapalbhati should be done after asana or neti, but just before concentration or meditation. It should not be practised at night, as it will cause difficulty sleeping.

Experienced practitioners with a strong and pure body can do this practice for hours at a time, but in general not more than ten to twenty rounds are recommended. Beginners should do two to three rounds only. After some weeks the number of rounds can be increased one at a time.

When is kapalbhati contra-indicated?

Swami Niranjanananda: If any feelings of unwellness are experienced, the practice should be stopped. It should not be practised in extremely hot weather, or when one is dehydrated, or suffering from irritability or anger. Although this practice can be adapted so that it is helpful during labour, it is not recommended during pregnancy without expert guidance.

Kapalbhati should not be undertaken by people suffering from high blood pressure, heart problems, ulcers, fever, constipation, hernia, anger or excessive restlessness.

What are the health benefits of practising kapalbhati?

Swami Sivananda: Kapalbhati cleanses the respiratory system and nasal passages, and removes spasm in the bronchial tubes. Consequently asthma is relieved and may be cured in the course of time. Tuberculosis may be cured by this practice. Impurities of the blood are thrown out. The apices of the lungs receive proper oxygenation and thereby do not afford a suitable breeding ground for bacteria.

The lungs are well developed by this practice. Carbon dioxide is largely eliminated, and the tissues and cells absorb a large quantity of oxygen. The heart functions properly. The circulatory and respiratory systems are toned, and the practitioner enjoys good health.

What are the general effects of kapalbhati on the body and mind?

Swami Satyananda: Kapalbhati is an excellent practice that purifies the frontal part of the brain, massages the abdominal organs and improves respiration.

Kapalbhati is also a powerful method of waking up the mind. The frontal lobes of the brain are cleared by speeding up the blood flow. At a more subtle level it also stimulates pranic flow in the same region. Therefore, if one has a lot of mental work to complete but feels tired, the mind can be energized and made alert with a few rounds of kapalbhati. It can be used to energize the mind for mental work when one feels tired, and to remove sleepiness early in the morning. It is an ideal practice to do immediately before commencing meditation techniques.

How does kapalbhati benefit the respiratory system?

Swami Satyananda: Kapalbhati benefits the respiratory system as it cleans out the lungs and improves their elasticity, resulting in more efficient exchange of oxygen and carbon dioxide.

Kapalbhati should certainly be practised by those suffering from respiratory ailments such as bronchitis and tuberculosis. Those who suffer from asthma and emphysema will, from habit and necessity, use forceful exhalation to expel air from the lungs. This tends to induce severe muscular tiredness. Kapalbhati, practised at times other than during an attack, may be useful in making respiratory muscles stronger, as well as improving the general tone of the lungs.

Why does kapalbhati energize the brain?

Swami Satyananda: Normal breathing is characterized by active contraction of only the inspiratory muscles, such as the diaphragm and the external intercostals; expiration occurs passively on the cessation of this contraction of the internal intercostals. Kapalbhati reverses this process: exhalation is active and inhalation is passive. This induces a reversal in the flow of the nerve impulses to and from the brain, bringing about stimulation and awakening of the brain centres. This is one reason for the brain-stimulating effect of kapalbhati, at least on a physiological basis. It should be noted that the expiratory muscles usually only come into action when there is obstruction to respiration, or when there is a great need of extra oxygen in the system.

Does the forced exhalation in kapalbhati have a direct effect on the brain?

Swami Satyananda: The effects of kapalbhati and bhastrika are similar, but due to the forced and longer exhalation, kapalbhati affects the brain differently. In his book, *Pranayama: The Yoga of Breathing*, Andre van Lysebeth describes a physiological phenomenon in which, during normal inhalation, the fluid around the brain is compressed causing the brain to contract slightly. With exhalation this cerebrospinal fluid is decompressed and the brain slightly expands. This is the mechanical influence of the respiratory cycle on the brain itself. Forced exhalation in kapalbhati increases the massaging effect on the brain by enhancing the decompression effect on every exhalation.

The average number of breaths being fifteen per minute, the brain is compressed and decompressed that many times, but in kapalbhati, one is breathing fifty to one hundred times, stimulating the brain three to seven times more than normal per round. Kapalbhati also expels more carbon dioxide and other waste gases from the cells and lungs than normal breathing.

What is the effect of kapalbhati on the pancha pranas?

Swami Niranjanananda: From the point of view of the pancha pranas, the role of prana (the active inhalation) and apana (the passive exhalation) are reversed, reducing samana, which on the mental level means a reduction in the activity of vrittis, or mental oscillations. This can be experienced during kapalbhati. At the same time the powerful upward flow created by the whole breathing attitude stimulates udana in the head and neck, which is in keeping with the meaning of the term 'kapalbhati'.

Does kapalbhati help prepare the sadhaka for the safe awakening of kundalini?

Swami Niranjanananda: Hatha yogis believe that ida and pingala nadis are purified by doing kapalbhati. In kundalini yoga it is said that at times one nadi flows while at other times the other nadi flows.

In general, the flow of breath in the nostrils, the *swara*, changes every ninety minutes. It alternates between the right nostril, which is associated with pingala nadi, and the left nostril, which is associated with ida nadi. When sushumna flows, prana moves freely through both nostrils at the same time. Only rarely do both nadis flow simultaneously, but it can be experienced if there is awareness of the breathing process. However, when the flow of the breath is equal in both nostrils, it still cannot be assumed that both ida and pingala nadis are free from disorders; an equal flow of air in both nostrils just happens from time to time.

It has also been said in kundalini yoga that if a practitioner does not have control over the swara and nadis, then pure, stainless kundalini, free from any disorder, could rise through nadis that are disordered and impure. If kundalini starts rising through ida or pingala nadi the person will begin to have certain experiences such as extreme dullness or excitability, depending on the state of the nadi and which nadi is involved. Without sufficient preparation of body, mind and prana, sometimes the person may even become mad, losing body consciousness. However, if the cleansing process has been done properly, the rising of kundalini will be through the sushumna passage.

How does the practice of kapalbhati assist in awakening ajna chakra?

Swami Niranjanananda: It is not kapalbhati which awakens ajna, but the reaction which takes place when one is able to perform a pranayama practice correctly that helps to awaken various chakras. Kapalbhati stimulates the nerves; they in turn activate the nadis, which then activate the pranas; the pranas are attracted towards the region in the nervous system where activity is taking place, which in kapalbhati is the forehead.

There are moments when the body, mind and prana all reach their peak at the same time, like the biorhythms which are calculated from the date of birth. According to the yogic concept, there are physical, mental and pranic biorhythms. When these three waves reach a certain point, there is harmony in the different koshas. This harmony is experienced in the form of a clear mind, thought and expression; increased nervous, emotional and mental energies; good health, physical fitness and mental relaxation. The biorhythms undergo many changes in the course of daily activities. Knowledge of these rhythms at the time of kapalbhati practice makes one deeply aware of the pranic and mental states. Kapalbhati helps to control the mental state by influencing the physical level, by altering the experiences, the input and output of the nervous system and the brain, and speeding up the metabolism.

In the context of hatha yoga, kapalbhati is practised to achieve a totally one-pointed state of mind. For the sake of understanding, the practice of kapalbhati may be compared to the state of pratyahara. In *pratyahara* one tries to divert the mind from external distractions and focus it at one point, and then in the practice of *dharana* one tries to intensify the concentration. In kapalbhati, like pratyahara, effort is made to relax the dissipation of the annamaya, manomaya and pranamaya koshas. The aim of kapalbhati is to awaken ajna chakra.

How does kapalbhati prepare one for the practice of meditation?

Swami Satyananda: Kapalbhati is one of the best preparatory techniques for meditative practice. It empties the mind of thoughts, emotional feelings and excessive visions. It induces a tranquil, receptive state of mind. At the same time, it energizes the mind so one is not overcome by sleep while sitting for meditation. Experience has shown that the ideal meditation practice to follow kapalbhati is chidakasha dharana.

What is the difference between hatha yoga and raja yoga kapalbhati?

Swami Satyananda: There are two ways of practising kapalbhati. The method of a hatha yogi is to simply expel the breath with force, whereas a raja yogi takes his awareness to *chidakasha*, the mind space, after the final expulsion. This additional practice removes certain cerebral tensions. Just as an expeller removes bad air from a room, even so the brain is shaken by the process of kapalbhati.

SURYA BHEDA PRANAYAMA: THE VITALITY STIMULATING BREATH

What is surya bheda pranayama?

Swami Satyananda: *Surya* is 'the sun' and it also refers to pingala nadi. *Bheda* has three meanings: 'secret', 'discrimination' and 'to pierce'. In this pranayama pingala nadi is activated by breathing in through the right nostril. Surya bheda pierces pingala and activates prana shakti in this nadi. *Hatha Yoga Pradipika* (2:48–49) describes the practice:

> *Aasane sukhade yogee badhvaa chaivaasanam tatah;*
> *Dakshanaadyaa samaakrishya bahihstham pavanam shanaih.*
>
> *Aakeshaadaanakhaagraachcha nirodhaavadhi kumbhayet;*
> *Tatah shanaih savyanaadyaa rechayetpavanam shanaih.*

Sitting comfortably, the yogi should become fixed in his posture and slowly breathe the air in through the right nostril. (48)

Retention should then be held until the breath diffuses to the roots of the hair and tips of the nails. Then slowly exhale through the left nostril. (49)

Surya bheda can also be practised by inhaling and exhaling through the right nostril only. However, when one only breathes through the right nostril, ida nadi and the functions of the left nostril are shut off. By exhaling through the left nostril there is a release of energy and any impurities that remain in ida. By inhaling through the right nostril the prana is drawn into pingala, and by retaining the breath after inhalation, the prana is kept in pingala.

If pingala nadi naturally predominates during the day, it is not advisable to practise this pranayama. When pingala flows, the mind and senses are extroverted, the left brain hemisphere functions, the sympathetic nervous system is active and the body is heated. Pingala should not be made to function excessively, it should be in harmony with the functioning of ida.

Unlike nadi shodhana pranayama, which balances the breath and brain hemispheres, surya bheda predominantly works on half the system. It stimulates the sympathetic nervous system and decreases the parasympathetic functions. Of course, this pranayama should only be done on an empty stomach, and it should only be done on the instructions of the guru.

What are the effects of surya bheda pranayama?

Swami Niranjanananda: Yogis and yogic scientists believe that the right nostril is connected with the sympathetic nervous system. When an activity is performed time and again with the right nostril, the sympathetic activity and rate of metabolism in the body are enhanced, causing changes to take place in the body.

This practice counteracts imbalances of the *vata dosha*, or wind element. It stimulates and awakens the pranic energy by activating pingala nadi and increasing extroversion and dynamism, enabling physical activities to be performed more effectively and efficiently. It is especially recommended for those who are dull and lethargic or who find it difficult to communicate with the external world. It makes the mind more alert and perceptive and is an excellent pre-meditation pranayama. Surya bheda is also useful in the treatment of low blood pressure, infertility and worms.

In *Gheranda Samhita* (5:69), the benefits of surya bheda pranayama are given:

Kumbhakah sooryabhedastu jaraamrityuvinaashakah;
Bodhayetkundaleem shaktim dehaanalavivardhanam;
Iti te kathitam chandam sooryabhedanamuttamam.

This pranayama, surya bheda, is the destroyer of old age and death. It awakens kundalini and the fire inside the body is activated. O Chanda, I have narrated to you the best pranayama known as surya bheda.

Addressing the king, Sage Gheranda draws his attention to this pranayama by saying it keeps away old age and death. It awakens kundalini shakti. It activates *agni*, meaning the fire or temperature in the body. Practising this pranayama can cause the body to overheat, which is beneficial during winter. Surya bheda is also useful for externalizing the consciousness in people who are depressed or introverted.

What is the effect of surya bheda pranayama on the brain?

Swami Satyananda: Surya bheda pranayama means 'piercing the sun'. By the very name of this pranayama, the left nostril is completely out of the picture, because the right nostril is associated with pingala nadi, which represents the dynamic energy of the sun.

There is another pranayama in hatha yoga known as chandra bheda pranayama. *Chandra bheda pranayama* means 'piercing the moon'. In that pranayama, the solar nadi is out of the picture.

From a scientific rather than a traditional point of view, when pranayama is practised, something happens to the brain. Scientific research has done a lot of work on the effect of pranayama through alternate nostrils. This research shows that when one breathes through the right nostril, the left hemisphere of the brain is immediately, within a moment, activated, influenced, affected. It does not take five minutes, it does not even take three minutes. Starting with the left nostril, the influence immediately takes place.

Now, when practising surya bheda pranayama, what is the purpose? The purpose is to activate, to awaken, to create an effect in the left hemisphere of the brain, not the right. The right must be excluded! If someone wants to include the right hemisphere of the brain, then why practise surya bheda? Practise nadi shodhana! In nadi shodana pranayama, there is an alternating impact on the right and left hemispheres due to the alternation of the breath through each nostril.

Surya bheda is practised to exclude the right hemisphere of the brain, for the time being. The practitioner does not want any effect to take place in the right hemisphere of the brain. Surya bheda pranayama is exclusively connected, related, and associated with the right nostril and the left hemisphere of the brain. It is referred to in the *Yoga Chudamani Upanishad* (v.97):

Sphuratprajvala sajjvaalaa poojuam aadityamandalam;
Dhyaatvaa hridi shitam yogee praanayaame sukhee bhavet.

At the time of pranayama, the yogi should meditate in the heart on the prescribed zone of the sun, which is blazing brightly. Having established this state, he should be happy.

What is the effect of surya bheda pranayama on the doshas, or humours of the body?

Swami Satyananda: In *Hatha Yoga Pradipika* (2:50), Yogi Swatmarama says that surya bheda eliminates imbalance of *vata*, the wind dosha:

Kapaalashodhanam vaatadoshaghnam krimidoshahyat;
Punahpunaridam kaaryam sooryabhedanamuttamam.

Surya bheda is excellent for purifying the cranium, destroying imbalances of the wind dosha and eliminating worms. It should be done again and again.

It also balances the other two doshas, *kapha*, mucus and *pitta*, bile. Stimulation of the sympathetic nervous system and pingala nadi removes dullness from the body and mind, and the heat produced through the practice burns up impurities in the body.

What precautions should be observed by those practising surya bheda pranayama?

Swami Niranjanananda: Never practise surya bheda prana-yama after eating as it will interfere with the natural flow

211

of energy associated with digestion. This pranayama may cause imbalance in the breathing cycle if performed for more than thirty minutes. Jalandhara and moola bandhas should be practised separately for some weeks or months before combining them in this pranayama practice.

Surya bheda pranayama should not be practised when suffering from external heat, boils, fever or constipation. People suffering from heart disease, hypertension, hyper-thyroid, peptic ulcer, anxiety, anger or epilepsy should not practise this pranayama.

Surya bheda is a most powerful pranayama and should only be performed under expert guidance.

PLAVINI: THE INUNDATING BREATH

What is plavini pranayama?

Swami Satyananda: *Plavana* means 'to float'. According to the hatha yoga texts, plavini pranayama enables one to float on water. It is an unusual form of pranayama which is similar to vatsara dhauti, except the air is retained in the stomach and intestines and not expelled immediately. It is described in *Hatha Yoga Pradipika* (2:70):

> *Antah pravartitodaaramaarutaapooritodarah;*
> *Payasyagaadhe'pi sukhaatplavate padmapatravat.*

> The inner part of the abdomen being completely filled with air, one can float like a lotus leaf on water.

This pranayama is rarely taught and little has ever been written about it. It is a practice that is generally handed down from guru to disciple.

9

Advanced Pranayamas

PRANAYAMA AND BANDHAS

What are bandhas?

Swami Niranjanananda: The word *bandha* means to 'hold', 'tighten' or 'lock'. These definitions describe the physical action involved in the bandha practices and their effect on the pranic body. Whereas mudras redirect prana by linking up certain circuits in the pranamaya kosha, bandhas redirect and store it by blocking the flow in certain areas of the body, thus forcing it to flow or accumulate in other areas. During the practices, certain parts of the body are contracted. This action also massages, stimulates and influences the muscles, organs, glands and nerves associated with that specific area.

One gains maximum benefit from pranayama when it is practised with the bandhas. When breath retention is practised in pranayama, bandhas should be performed.

What are the four bandhas?

Swami Satyananda: There are four bandhas. When the perineum is contracted, that is *moola bandha*. When the abdomen is contracted, that is *uddiyana bandha*. When the chin is locked against the throat, that is *jalandhara* bandha. The fourth bandha is *maha bandha*, a combination of the previous three. These three bandhas are important for their

213

effect on the lungs, the heart, the nervous system, and finally, the brain.

Why are the bandhas used when practising pranayama?

Swami Satyananda: According to hatha yoga, the practice of pranayama should be integrated with the three bandhas: jalandhara bandha, uddiyana bandha, and moola bandha.

When pranayama is practised, the pranas in the lower region of the body are stimulated, but there needs to be a means of forcing the pranic energy up. Somehow, a negative force has to be created which will push the pranic energy up through the spinal cord. For this reason pranayama should be practised in coordination with specific bandhas.

The three bandhas which are incorporated into the practice of pranayama create a negative force like the ejecting force used to extract water from a well. There are two forces used for pumping water – the sucking force and the ejecting force. When pranayama is practised with the bandhas, an ejecting force is put into action.

Prana is generated in the lower region of the body by pranayama; in order to focus and then redirect it up to the brain, one must practise moola bandha, then jalandhara bandha and finally uddiyana bandha. Moola bandha is contraction of the perineum, uddiyana bandha is lifting the diaphragm up and jalandhara bandha is the locking of the chin against the sternum. Prana is then conducted to the brain with the help of the subtle pranic circulatory system.

Are the bandhas always practised with breath retention?

Swami Satyananda: When the breath is retained, it is important to hold the three bandhas. Without practising and perfecting the three bandhas, kumbhaka should not be practised. The three bandhas are named jalandhara bandha, uddiyana bandha, and moola bandha. When the breath is held in, then jalandhara and moola bandha must be practised, and when the lungs are emptied, and the breath is held out, the three bandhas are done. This is called *maha bandha*.

214

What is the role of mudras and bandhas in pranayama?

Swami Satyananda: Pranayama actually involves the practice of breath control in combination with bandhas and mudras. Pranayama should be practised with bandhas, in the proper sitting posture and with the appropriate mudra. Either *shambhavi mudra*, focusing the gaze on the eyebrow centre, or *nasikagra mudra*, focusing on the nosetip should be used.

Without bandhas, pranayama is incomplete. Either the three bandhas: jalandhara, uddiyana and moola bandha, should be done together or in different combinations. This is described in *Hatha Yoga Pradipika* (2:45–46):

Poorakaante tu kartavyo bandho jaalandharaabhidhah;
Kumbhakaante rechakaadau kartavyastooddiyaanakah.

Adhastaatkunchanenaashu kanthasankochane krite;
Madhye pashchimataanena syaatpraano brahmanaadigah.

At the end of inhalation, jalandhara bandha is done. At the end of kumbhaka and beginning of exhalation, uddiyana bandha is done.

By contracting the perineum, contracting the throat and drawing the abdomen up, the prana flows into the brahma nadi.

According to Yogi Swatmarama, uddiyana should be done after retention and at the beginning of *rechaka*, exhalation. Once exhalation is complete, jalandhara bandha should be done and uddiyana fully employed. Uddiyana bandha is only practised with external retention, or *bahiranga kumbhaka*, as then the stomach and lungs are completely empty and the abdomen can easily be drawn in and up.

Moola bandha or contraction of the muscles of the perineal body or cervix can be done with either *antaranga*, inner retention, or bahiranga kumbhaka. After inhalation, jalandhara and moola bandha are practised together, and after exhalation the three bandhas are performed. When the three bandhas are practised in combination, this is called

215

maha bandha. However, in certain pranayama practices the three bandhas cannot be done together. For example, it is inappropriate to perform uddiyana bandha in moorchha pranayama.

Though the bandhas are used in pranayama they are considered as separate practices. Bandhas are powerful practices that generate and accumulate prana in specific parts of the physical and subtle bodies; they are essential in the practices to awaken the chakras and sushumna nadi

When and how are bandhas introduced into pranayama?

Swami Niranjanananda: The aim of pranayama initially is to activate the pranas through breath control, and later on through the practices of mudra and bandha. Therefore, mudra and bandha are incorporated in the later stages of pranayama. Initially, when dealing with the normal breathing process, there is no practise of bandha with pranayama.

For example, in nadi shodhana one begins with simple breathing in and out through the nostrils. Gradually the duration of inhalation and exhalation is lengthened, and then ratios of inner and outer retention are added. As one progresses further, bandhas are incorporated into the practice of nadi shodhana. After inhalation, jalandhara bandha and moola bandha are practised while holding the breath inside, then after releasing the bandhas, the practitioner breathes out and practises the three bandhas: jalandhara, uddiyana and moola, while holding the breath out. In this way, nadi shodhana is combined with bandhas

What sitting asana is used while practising pranayama with bandhas?

Swami Satyananda: These bandhas should be practised in the two prescribed asanas. The best one is siddhasana for males and siddha yoni asana for females. *Padmasana*, the lotus posture, can also be used. Why is this important? During pranayama the body is an electrical pole. If there is no circuit, then the energy is going to be lost through the earth

216

connection. Therefore, there is a scientific reason for using these postures.

The left foot carries the cool energy and the right foot carries the hot energy. The cool energy and the hot energy are known as the negative and the positive energy. There must be a complete circuit of both. This is not necessary for a beginner. But for those who want to go further in pranayama, lotus posture or siddhasana or siddha yoni asana are imperative.

When the body produces more energy, it can leave through the earth connection. That leakage must be avoided. That is why the proper asanas and bandhas are necessary in pranayama.

How are the prana vayus influenced by practising bandhas during pranayama?

Swami Satyananda: One gains the maximum benefits from pranayama when the bandhas are practised with breath retention. Without bandhas, pranayama is of no use. A scientist generates energy then captures it. He accumulates it, and then sends it through the cables to the transformers and to people's rooms and to factories. Nature is creating energy all the time, but man does not know how to tame it. In the same way, when pranayama is practised, energy is created, a force is created and this force is in the cerebrospinal system, in the centre of the spine.

Pranayama stimulates the flow of prana and the bandhas control the flow and direct it to the required areas. *Prana*, as in the vital energy between the larynx and diaphragm, is an evolutionary force, a non-material force; it is in the physical body and it is in the universe. *Apana*, meaning the vital energy in the lower part of the body, is an instinctive force or a material force. In this physical body these two forces are to be brought to the central zone in the navel and that can be done only through the practice of uddiyana bandha.

When moola bandha is performed, the apana is forced to flow upwards. When jalandhara is performed, the prana is forced to flow downwards and unite with apana. When prana

217

and apana unite it is a fantastic experience which generates vitality and helps to awaken kundalini.

Generally the tendency of the force is to go down. The general tendency of energy and force is to dissipate. In science it is said that any energy, any electromagnetic energy or gravitational force or electrical energy has a natural tendency to dissipate, and in this physical body that is also the tendency. Therefore, the natural tendency towards dissipation must be obstructed by the practice of uddiyana bandha in synchronization with pranayama practices.

What is the relationship between bandhas, kumbhaka and consciousness?

Swami Satyananda: According to yogic scripture, control of muscles and nerves controls the breath. Control of breath controls consciousness. Bandhas are a means of extending control over breathing and are thus a means to extend one's knowledge and control over consciousness.

The breathing rate and depth is said to be affected by: states of consciousness, disease, atmospheric conditions, thoughts, exercise and emotions. Research has shown that in states of tension and fear respiration becomes short and shallow, while in states of relaxation, people take long deep breaths.

When bandhas are performed in conjunction with pranayama, contraction of the muscles takes place simultaneously with kumbhaka (internal or external breath retention). The physical lock or contraction is applied and at the same time the breath is also arrested or immobilized. As a consequence the consciousness is arrested, stopping the flow between the polar opposites of inhalation and exhalation, birth and death, joy and sorrow, gain and loss.

Why is moola bandha used with kumbhaka?

Swami Satyananda: For maximum benefits moola bandha should be practised in conjunction with pranayama. This is because while pranayama stimulates and allows control of the flow of prana, the bandha directs it to required areas, thus preventing dissipation. In the context of pranayama, apana moves up with inhalation and prana moves down with exhalation, while a balance between inhalation and exhalation signifies the retention of breath which occurs spontaneously when prana and apana unite.

Moola bandha is used with kumbhaka as it helps to turn the apana upwards. In the beginning moola bandha should be practised with internal breath retention. Simultaneously the region of the perineum is contracted and pulled up towards the diaphragm. When the practitioner can perform moola bandha while holding the breath inside, without the slightest strain or discomfort, then he should attempt the more difficult practice of moola bandha with external breath retention which has a more powerful effect.

What are some examples of perfected kumbhaka?

Swami Niranjanananda: Very few people in the world have, through their own effort, actually awakened the prana shakti in their body. One example is Swami Nadabrahmananda, a disciple of Swami Sivananda. When he came to the ashram, Swami Sivananda told him, "Perfect pranayama." This swami reached a level of competency in pranayama where he could actually hold his breath without breathing in or out for one hour.

He was also a tabla player and playing the tabla is physically exerting. Research was conducted by Dr Elmer Green at the Menninger Foundation, USA, using three identical airtight glass chambers. In one chamber they lit a candle, and the candle went out after three minutes, meaning that the oxygen was finished. In another chamber they had a monkey, and the monkey fell down unconscious after about ten minutes, which meant that there was a very high concentration of carbon dioxide. In the third chamber they put Swami Nadabrahmananda.

They had put wax all over his body, plugged all the orifices and attached electrodes to his body. Inside

219

the chamber he had to play the tabla while practising kumbhaka, and he did that for one hour. During this period everybody was convinced that there was not even a particle of oxygen going into his body. The research was done under such tight conditions that there was no possibility of having any fresh air.

When I questioned Swami Nadabrahmanandaji about how he was able to retain his breath for one hour, he said to me, "I hold the breath in my manipura and from manipura that prana shakti is distributed." He was describing to me the process of prana vidya, because this is another technique of yoga, much more advanced then pranayamas. The aspirant is guided to generate prana shakti in mooladhara, store it in manipura and distribute it through ajna: this is the system of prana vidya. The process being described by Swami Nadabrahmanandaji was exactly the process of prana vidya and he said, "After I had perfected my pranayamas, Swami Sivanandaji instructed me to perfect prana vidya and because of this I can stop my respiration today for one hour in a very comfortable way without any side effects." Swami Nadabrahmananda died at the age of ninety-eight.

Another person whom I have seen hold the breath, and who was submerged in water, was Pilot Baba. These people had perfected the art of pranayama.

Pranayama leads to perception of prana shakti and absorption of prana shakti from the environment. The more advanced practice of prana vidya actually taps into the source of prana shakti within the body at the level of the chakras. Again, in this practice of prana vidya, one is taught to have certain experiences by regulating the breath and to intensify those experiences through further breath regulation, visualization, concentration, and the experience of heat and lightness. With the prana vidya practice the chakras are also activated, more specifically the three chakras mooladhara, manipura and ajna.

In kundalini yoga these three chakras are responsible for the awakening and direction of prana shakti. This is the indication which we receive from the practice of the three bandhas as well. Moola bandha controls mooladhara chakra and it reverses the flow of prana shakti upwards. Uddiyana bandha controls manipura chakra and jalandhara bandha creates pressure at ajna chakra. Prana vidya combined with the three bandhas can definitely help in producing the subtle pranic energy in the body.

THE PRACTICE OF KUMBHAKA: RETENTION OF THE BREATH

What is kumbhaka?

Swami Sivananda: *Kumbhaka* means cessation of the breath. It is when there is neither expiration nor inspiration and the body is motionless, remaining still in one state.

Kumbhaka is of two kinds, namely sahita and kevala. That which is coupled with inhalation and exhalation is termed *sahita*. That which is devoid of these is called *kevala*, alone. When kumbhaka occurs without exhalation and inhalation, and is unconditioned by place, time and number, that kumbhaka is called absolute and pure – it is kevala kumbhaka.

Why do yogis practise breath regulation?

Swami Sivananda: There is neither rhythm nor harmony in the breathing of worldly-minded people. A yogi practices regulation of breath to establish harmony. When the breath is regulated, when there is harmony, the breath will move rhythmically within the nostrils.

The fruit of regulation of breath is *kumbhaka*, retention of the breath. The breath stops by itself when *kevala kumbhaka*, absolute and pure retention of breath, follows. The mind spontaneously becomes steady, and *samadhi*, the superconscious state, supervenes. Regulation of breath, and kumbhaka, are of tremendous help in the practice of concentration and meditation.

221

Why is it said that breath retention is pranayama?

Swami Satyananda: Pranayama is a difficult practice. In order to charge the brain with sufficient prana, it must be practised systematically. Pranayama is usually considered to be the practice of controlled inhalation and exhalation combined with retention. There are many varieties of pranayama, such as nadi shodhana, bhramari, kapalbhati, bhastrika and ujjayi.

These are not actually pranayamas, they are varieties of the practice. Technically speaking, pranayama is only retention. In the traditional yoga texts it is clearly indicated that retention of the breath is pranayama. They say that the gap between inhalation and exhalation is pranayama. Sage Patanjali defines pranayama in this way in the *Yoga Sutras* (2:49):

> *Tasminsati shvaasaprashvaasayorgativichchhedaha praanaayaamaha*

> The asana having been done, pranayama is the cessation of the movement of inhalation and exhalation.

Inhalation and exhalation are methods of inducing retention. Retention is most important because it allows a longer period for assimilation of prana, just as it allows more time for the exchange of gases – oxygen and carbon dioxide – in the cells.

Retention of breath is done at two points. When the lungs have been filled, *antar kumbhaka* is practised by holding the breath in, and when the lungs are emptied, *bahir kumbhaka* is practised by holding the breath out. Both forms of kumbhaka are important and are so powerful that they can completely rejuvenate the brain. That is pranayama.

Why is breath retention the most important stage of pranayama?

Swami Satyananda: Sage Patanjali says that retention of breath after expiration removes the obstacles to yoga. Yoga is the union of the two poles of energy within us. In mundane awareness these poles are separate from each other. In transcendental awareness these poles come closer together, and during retention the poles come closest together. Breath retention must be developed in order to stop the fluctuations of the brain and mind so that a more expansive type of experience can develop.

What is the difference between kumbhaka in hatha yoga and in raja yoga?

Swami Satyananda: When one breathes in and then breathes out there is a gap; when one goes to this door and then returns from this door there is a point where one stops – that is the point of return and that is the point where one stopped, only for a split second. Stop there for more time, and that is called kumbhaka, which means the breath does not go in and the breath does not go out.

There are two types of kumbhaka. One kumbhaka is done through practice; the breath is taken in and stopped, the breath is exhaled and stopped. The other kumbhaka occurs when one has gone into meditation through practising kumbhaka as just described, and the breath stops spontaneously; it may stop at the end of inspiration or it may stop at the end of expiration or it may stop in between – it has not been consciously stopped. When the mind stops, the breath stops or when the breath stops, the mind stops. This is the central teaching about pranayama in the *Hatha Yoga Pradipika*.

Therefore yogis practise pranayama differently – the hatha yogi practises kumbhaka voluntarily; he trains himself to stop the breath and thus he stops his mind. The raja yogi does not do this; he does just a little pranayama, that's all; he does not do special practice of pranayama; he does simple and normal practice of pranayama. Then he concentrates, he meditates and when concentration takes place, the breath stops, as the prana and the mind are interconnected. The breath and the brain are interrelated, and it has also been observed that when one does kumbhaka, extra electrical impulses are registered through certain centres in the spinal cord.

What happens during breath retention?

Swami Niranjanananda: Sage Patanjali describes four types of pranayama in the *Yoga Sutras*. Two involve internal breath retention and two involve external retention. Internal breath retention is easy and does not place much strain on the body. Most people can hold the breath inside for twenty or twenty-five seconds without strain. When air is inside the lungs, the exchange of oxygen and carbon dioxide between the air and the blood continues for a short time.

External breath retention, however, is more difficult. When the breath is held out, the flow of blood to the heart is decreased, as pressure in the chest is high at the end of exhalation. Additionally, there is a lack of oxygen available to the blood in the lungs. These factors cause the heart rate to increase to try to pump an adequate amount of oxygen around the body. However, the fast heart rate uses up more oxygen and produces more waste carbon dioxide. Thus, after only a short period there is a need to breathe in again.

Through the medium of pranayama both the nervous system and prana shakti can be balanced. Internal and external breath retention are practised to create different states. In hatha yoga and kundalini yoga, perfection of breath retention is associated with awakening of the chakras and kundalini.

When does breath retention occur in daily life?

Swami Sivananda: The porter carrying heavy bags of rice or wheat at the wharf instinctively fills his lungs with air and practises unconscious retention of breath until the bag is lifted onto his back. This retention of breath augments his strength and vitality. It immediately provides him with an abundance of energy. It induces great concentration of mind. When one crosses a small rivulet by jumping over it, when one practises long jump and high jump and other exercises at the parallel bar and trapeze, retention of breath is practised instinctively.

How can kumbhaka be developed?

Swami Sivananda: The period of retention is gradually increased. In the beginning a time unit for inhalation, retention and exhalation must be observed. The time unit and the proper ratio come by themselves. One may start with four seconds in the first week, try eight seconds in the second week, twelve seconds in the third week and so on. Eventually full capacity will be reached. In the advanced stages, the mind should not be distracted with counting. The lungs will say when the required number is finished.

What is samaveta pranayama?

Swami Satyananda: The Sanskrit word *samaveta* means 'together'. Therefore samaveta pranayama is a practice where one breathes through both the nostrils. This might seem to be an obvious and inconsequential statement, but the practice is so named to distinguish it from other techniques of pranayama where the flow of air is directed in one nostril by physically or mentally preventing the flow in the other nostril. Samaveta involves gentle and gradual development of internal breath retention. Over a period of weeks the time of breath retention may slowly be increased from a second or so to a maximum of ten seconds.

In samaveta one starts by practising rhythmic yogic breathing for a while. Once this is established, the practitioner simply holds the breath in briefly at the end of inhalation. In the beginning this may be for only one second. Gradually the capacity for retention will increase. This should happen naturally, without any forcing. The breathing should be as slow as is comfortable.

This is an excellent practice to prepare the lungs for more advanced practices of pranayama. At the time of retention the amount of oxygen taken up by the blood and the amount of carbon dioxide which is discharged by the blood into the lungs is increased. When people breathe quickly and shallowly the exchange between the circulating blood and the lungs is quite small. The increased exchange during samaveta pranayama helps to revitalize the body and improve the health. It lays the groundwork for the practice of pranayama with kumbhaka.

Some people think that retention of breath is harmful, what do the yogic texts say?

Swami Satyananda: A lot of scientific studies have been done on the effect of retention on the brain, body, heart etc., and nothing negative has been shown. Therefore it cannot be said that retention has a negative effect on the aspirant. In the authentic yogic texts, the definition of pranayama is, 'retention of breath'. Therefore, if retention is not acceptable, the very science of pranayama has to be deleted from the yoga texts.

The authentic texts on pranayama are *Hatha Yoga Pradipika, Goraksha Samhita, Gheranda Samhita, Hatharatnavali* and *Sri Vijnana Bhairava Tantra*. They are considered to be the textbooks on hatha yoga in particular and pranayama in general. In these texts no such warnings are given. Therefore, these warnings are illogical and should be discarded. *Sri Vijnana Bhairava Tantra* (v. 25–27) speaks in detail of the importance of kumbhaka:

Maruto'ntar bahir vaapi viyadyugmaanivartanaat;
Bhairavyaa bhairavasyettham bhairavi vyajyate vapuh.

Na vrajen na vishechchhaktir marudroopaa vikaasite;
Nirvikalpatayaa madhye tayaa bhairavaroopataa.

Kumbhitaa rechitaa vaapi pooritaa yaa yadaa bhavet;
Tadante shaantanaamaasau shaktyaa shaantah prakaashate.

When the ingoing pranic air and outgoing pranic air are both restrained in their space from their (respective points of) return, the essence of bhairava, which is not different from bhairavi, manifests. (25)

When shakti in the form of vayu or pranic air is still and does not move swiftly in a specific direction, there develops in the middle, through the state of nirvikalpa, the form of Bhairava. (26)

When kumbhaka takes place after pooraka or rechaka, then the shakti known as shanta is experienced and through that peace (the bhairava consciousness) is revealed. (27)

Why is it advisable to proceed slowly in the practice of antar kumbhaka?

Swami Satyananda: Though antar kumbhaka is a seemingly simple and straightforward practice, it does have vast repercussions on the body and mind. One must be alert to any adverse reactions. These can take a variety of forms from excessive spots on the skin to the inability to sleep.

When spots appear, the kumbhaka is rapidly purging the body of inherent impurities. Due to the rapidity the poisons cause numerous spots to erupt on the skin as they are expelled. If this happens the practice of kumbhaka should be reduced or even stopped for a short time to allow the body to cleanse more slowly. If insomnia develops, kumbhaka is in a sense overcharging the body and mind above its normal level of activity and the practice should be reduced or stopped for some time. There are many other possible adverse reactions. Be alert to them and if necessary seek the advice and guidance of a competent yoga teacher.

The reason for any kind of adverse reaction is generally too much practice in the early stages. One should be moderate in the time spent daily doing pranayama, especially kumbhaka. For the first six months no more than ten minutes should be done. If a person wants to do more and their constitution is adequate then it will probably be all right and there may be great benefits. One should always consult an experienced teacher if there is any doubt about practices.

It is emphasized that the duration of antar kumbhaka should be slowly increased without any strain so that the body mechanisms are slowly accustomed to the new level of functioning. The first stages of nadi shodhana pranayama should definitely be practised for at least a month before attempting serious practice of antar kumbhaka.

What effect does antar kumbhaka have on the pranic and mental bodies?

Swami Satyananda: Antar kumbhaka has a marked influence on the flow of prana throughout the pranic body. Since there is a close relationship between the pranic body and the mind, antar kumbhaka in turn allows one to gain some control over the mind. Unfortunately, most people have a mind that is in a continual state of disturbance and fluctuation. Antar kumbhaka slows down the tumultuous mind and transforms it into a state of peaceful one-pointedness, a prerequisite for the state of meditation. The pranic effect of antar kumbhaka is described in *Yoga Chudamani Upanishad* (v.100):

> *Praano dehasthito yaavadapaanam tu nirundhayet;*
> *Ekahvaasamayee maatraa oordhvaadho gagane sthitih.*

> As long as prana remains in the body, apana should be retained, so that the quantity drawn in one breath remains and moves up and down in hridayakasha.

How important are the ratios used in pranayama?

Swami Satyananda: Ratio in pranayama is important, deep breathing is not important. In relation to pranayama, the ratio between inhalation, retention and exhalation must be maintained in order to have balance, to have coordination between the heart, the nervous system, the lungs and the brain. Ratio in pranayama is described in *Yoga Chudamani Upanishad* (v. 103–104):

> *Poorakam dvaadasham kuryaat kumbhakam shodasham bhavet;*
> *Rechakam dasha chomaarah praanaayaamah sa uchyate.*

> *Adhame dvaadashaa maatraa madhyama dvigunaa mataa;*
> *Uttama triguna proktaa pranaayaamasya nirnayah.*

The inhalation should be practised to the count of twelve, retention to the count of sixteen and exhalation to the count of ten. This is called the Omkara pranayama. (103)

About pranayama it has been said that the lowest level is twelve counts, the middle level is double that or twenty-four counts, and the highest level is triple or thirty-six counts. (104)

The ratio depends on the aspirant. For some it could be 1:1:2:1 and for some it could be 1:2:2:1. For others it could even be 1:4:2:2. It depends on one's personal capacity and the extent of one's practice.

With this practice the consciousness is immediately affected. When the consciousness is affected, the veil is removed and light is experienced. This light is not the external light that one sees. This is the light in which one becomes free from all the sorrows of life. It is known as enlightenment. Therefore, in one's day-to-day practice, retention should be perfected.

Why is Gayatri mantra used as a way of counting durations in pranayama?

Swami Satyananda: Somehow the breath has to be counted during prayanama. In many yogic texts, it is suggested to clap one and snap one, but this is disturbing and cumbersome. Counting is also inaccurate. The most accurate way to count is mantra. One's personal mantra is not appropriate because it is not accurate. The mantra which is used for measuring the duration of the breath is *Gayatri* mantra.

Gayatri is a mantra of twenty-four syllables, and when it is repeated mentally, the practitioner completes one vital circle of the breath. Everybody has a different vital capacity. Some people take in less air and others take in more.

The twenty-four syllables of *Gayatri* mantra are: *Tat savitur varenyam, bhargo devasya dhi mahi, diyo yo naha prachodayat.* Gayatri mantra is equal in length to the ideal vital capacity.

229

Therefore, on inhalation one mentally says one *Gayatri* mantra. During internal breath retention, it is repeated once or twice, depending on capacity. On exhalation, it is repeated twice and when the breath is retained outside, it is said once.

Gayatri mantra is ideal, but it is not compulsory. Any other mantra can be used, however it is difficult to tell exactly how many repetitions will be equal to the vital capacity. That, one has to decide for oneself. It could be 2, 3, 4, 5, 6, 7, 8 – who knows? For this reason, one should learn *Gayatri* mantra.

Gayatri is not a personal mantra. *Gayatri* mantra is intended for pranayama. It relates to the breath. It is said that *Gayatri* is the pranic force, the life force. So, in order to use one's prana for concentration and meditation, practise *Gayatri* mantra with pranayama.

Gayatri is the sound which makes the mind free from the senses. One cannot meditate because the mind is in the clutches of the senses. The greatest disturbing factor in meditation is the senses. Like a postman, every now and then, these senses bring the news and when they bring the news, they disturb the mind. The mind has to be rendered free from the clutches of the senses, and that is the role of *Gayatri* mantra.

What symptoms indicate progress in the practice of kumbhaka?

Swami Satyananda: When practising kumbhaka, after perhaps one hour or so, if it feels like everything is becoming dark inside, that is a negative symptom. Sometimes it feels as if the inner space is becoming more and more enlightened. That is a positive symptom. Then there are other external symptoms, such as the smell of the body. Sometimes people have an awful smell coming from the body. This means kumbhaka is working on the catabolic process.

When kumbhaka is practised fat is burned from the body. In spite of that, the practitioner's glow is radiant. In *Hatha Yoga Pradipika* (2:19), this effect is described:

Yadaa tu naadeeshuddhih syaattathaa chihnaani baahyatah;
Kaayasya krishataa kaantistadaa jaayeta nishchitam.

When the nadis are purified, there are external symptoms. Success is definite when the body becomes thin and glows.

This is the proof that one's practice is working. *Yoga Chudamani Upanishad* (v.105) describes the effects of different levels of kumbhaka in pranayama:

Adhame sedajananam kampo bhavati madhyama;
Uttama sthaanamaapnoti tato vayum nirundhayet.

The lowest level causes perspiration. The middle level results in trembling of the body. At the highest level stability is achieved. Therefore, the breath should be retained.

These things should be discussed between the teacher and the pupil.

How is it possible for yogis to stop the breath and stay alive?

Swami Niranjanananda: A yogi who has perfected pranayama can hold the breath for an extended period of time without any ill effects and without dying. If someone comes and holds my nose and mouth and I cannot breath, in a few minutes I will have to say, "Hari Om Tat Sat, see you in the next life." But if I have been able to perfect pranayama, then no matter who holds my nose and mouth, I can continue to be alive for as long as I want, without breathing.

A famous example of this is Swami Nadabrahmananda, a disciple of Swami Sivananda who perfected the art of pranayama. He could hold his breath for forty-five minutes while performing strenuous activities such as playing tabla. Research demonstrating the importance of prana was conducted on him by Dr Elmer Green at the Menninger Foundation in the USA. Swami Nadabrahmananda was completely covered in wax, his nostrils, ears and all the openings of his body were plugged: there was no way a single particle of oxygen could enter his body. He was put in an airtight chamber where he started playing tabla. He did not breathe, but he played tabla very fast for forty-five minutes. When asked how he was able to do it, he simply said, "Nada kumbhaka; because of nada kumbhaka I was able to do this."

When Swami Satyananda was asked about it, he said, "Yes, it is possible that with the perfection of pranayama there is disassociation of the breath from prana." Once that occurs, whether one breathes or not is irrelevant; one can sit down under water for hours together without breathing and remain alive. This is an example of prana shakti. Therefore, the breath should not be equated with prana, or pranayama with breath exercises. Initially, however, control over the breath is needed in order to tap the source of prana shakti.

How does kumbhaka affect ajna chakra?

Swami Satyananda: The practices of shambhavi and of trataka strengthen ajna chakra, but kumbhaka, retention of the breath is the most important. When the breath is retained and the three bandhas are practised, this is kumbhaka. When kumbhaka takes place, ajna chakra automatically begins to wake up. Initially some people may feel various physical sensations at this point, but these are only important in relation to the fact that ajna chakra is operating.

What is the effect of kumbhaka on the kundalini?

Swami Satyananda: Kumbhaka is responsible for the awakening of kundalini. There are many ways in which one can awaken this potential power, such as through laya yoga and tantra yoga. Pranayama, however, is the most powerful method. If one is practising pranayama and heat is generated in the body, if pain is felt in the body, if restlessness comes, if there is a feeling of being completely lost in relation to experiences of the empirical world, if one begins to understand the sun and the moon and nature in a new way, why wonder at it? When kumbhaka changes the quality of the mind, it will definitely change the quality of one's perception. In *Hatha Yoga Pradipika* (2:43) it is said:

Tatsiddhahye vidhaanajnaashchitraankurvanti kumbhakaan;
Vichitra kumbhakaabhyaasaadvichitraam siddhimaapnuyaat.

By practising the various kumbhakas wondrous perfections are obtained. Those who are the knowers practise the various kumbhakas to accomplish them.

What are the signs of pranic awakening in advanced pranayama?

Swami Niranjanananda: Sage Gheranda describes pranayama practised without mantra, and its effects on the pranas. It is divided into three levels: *uttama,* the highest or advanced, *madhyama,* the medium or intermediate, and *adhama,* the lowest or beginners, based on counting. In *Gheranda Samhita* (5:54–56) it is written:

Praanaayaamo nirgarbhastu vinaa beejena jaayate;
Vaamajaanooparinyastam vaamapaanitalam bhramet;
Ekaadishataparyantam poorakumbhakarechakam.

Uttamaa vimshatirmaatraa madhyamaa shodashee smritaa;
Adhamaa dvaadashee maatraa praanaayaamaastridhaa smritaah.

Adhamaajjaayate gharmo merukampashcha madhyamaat;
Uttamaachcha bhoomityaagastrividham siddhilakshanam.

Nirgarbha pranayama is practised without bija mantras; the left hand moves on the left knee (to keep count) of the pranayama consisting of inhalation, retention and exhalation from one to one hundred. (54)

The highest pranayama has twenty counts, the medium sixteen and the lowest twelve. Thus pranayama has three wings. (55)

233

The lowest gives birth to heat or perspiration; through the middle count trembling of the body (especially the spine) is achieved, and by the highest, the practitioner is lifted up from the earth and travels in space. These three (experiences) should all be considered as symptoms of mastery. (56)

Different symptoms are observed, indicating that a particular stage has been perfected. If the body starts to sweat during adhama nirgarbha pranayama, this indicates that the ratio 12:48:24 has been perfected and awakening of the pranas is commencing.

The symptom of perfecting madhyama nirgarbha is the sensation of vibrations in the spinal cord. Vibrations in the spine take place for two reasons: firstly, when the pranas are awakened in the chakras and secondly, when kundalini is awakened and starts ascending in the upper chakras. With perfection of the count 16:64:32, the state of *pranotthana*, pranic awakening, has come, after which the body is ready for the awakening of the kundalini.

A person who has mastery over inhalation, retention and exhalation in the ratio of 20:80:40, must be able to exercise control over the breath, physical and internal uneasiness, mental anxiety and the state of the brain. On perfection of this *uttama pranayama*, then *bhoomi tyaga* is achieved, meaning the pranas are expanded, and in that state prana shakti awakens, making the body light so it becomes capable of leaving or rising above the earth.

KEVALA KUMBHAKA:
SPONTANEOUS RETENTION OF BREATH

What is kevala kumbhaka?

Swami Satyananda: There is a certain moment when prana and the mind interact and move together. When the mind is controlled the pranic forces stop and when the pranas are controlled the mind automatically stops. In yoga, this is known as *kevala kumbhaka*, automatic, spontaneous retention. The moment the mind ceases to function or is consumed in the point of concentration, automatically the breath must stop because in the brain these two activities are interconnected. Kevali pranayama, therefore, is important because it indicates that mental stability has been achieved.

The raja yogis first control the mind then stop the breath. Hatha yogis control the breath and thereby control the fluctuations of the mind. The moment the mind becomes active, the breath is also resurrected, because the mind and the breath are two companions. They live together, move together, fly together and die together. If the prana is resurrected, the mind is resurrected; if the mind is resurrected, the prana is resurrected. When kevala kumbhaka takes place allow it to happen without resisting because it culminates in the awakening.

What is the difference between sahita and kevala kumbhaka?

Swami Satyananda: When kumbhaka is practised with conscious effort it is called *sahita* or connected retention. When it happens by itself, without any apparent reason or association with either pooraka or rechaka, then it is *kevala* or unconnected, unsupported retention. Sahita pranayama influences the conscious and subconscious levels, namely the body, prana, mind and psyche. Kevala kumbhaka results in the awakening of the unconscious mind and body, and leads to a state beyond that. In *Hatha Yoga Pradipika* (2:71–72) it is said:

Praanaayaamastridhaa prokto rechapoorakakumbhakaih;
Sahitah kevalashcheti kumbhako dvividho matah.

Yaavatkevalasiddhih syaatsahitam taavadabhyaset;
Rechakam poorakam muktvaa sukham yadvaayudhaaranam.

Pranayama is said to be of three types: exhalation, inhalation and retention. Retention is again of two types: connected (sahita) and unconnected (kevala). (71)

Until kevala kumbhaka is perfected, sahita kumbhaka has to be practised. When (you are) freed of inhalation and exhalation, the breath (prana) is retained easily. (72)

The purpose of all pranayama practices is to create a perfectly still state in the body so that inhalation and exhalation stop with the cessation of pranic movement. Control of the breath, prana and body means control of the wavering tendencies or oscillations of the mind. All hatha yoga techniques eventually lead to this state of kevala kumbhaka, when prana and mind stop moving. In *Hatha Yoga Pradipika* (2:73–74) it is said:

Praanaayaamo'yamityuktah sa vai kevalakumbhakam;
Kumbhake kevale siddhe rechapoorakavarjite.

Na tasya durlabham kinchittrishu lokeshu vidyate;
Shaktah kevalakumbhena yatheshtam vaayudhaaranaat.

Perfection of isolated retention is freedom from inhalation and exhalation. This pranayama spoken of is verily kevala kumbhaka. (73)

Nothing in the three planes of existence is unobtainable for one who has mastery of kevala kumbhaka and can retain the breath as desired. (74)

The three planes are the conscious, subconscious and unconscious: *jagrat, swapna* and *sushupti*.

Sahita pranayama is divided into two divisions: *sagarbha*, with mantra repetition, and *nirgarbha*, without mantra repetition. Throughout the eight pranayama practices in *Hatha Yoga Pradipika* Yogi Swatmarama has not referred to mantra repetition, therefore all those practices are forms of nirgarbha pranayama. However, in the *Gheranda Samhita* and *Hatharatnavali* sagarbha is referred to.

236

What are the fruits of perfecting kevala kumbhaka?

Swami Sivananda: Such powers as that of roaming about in space unseen follow this kevala kumbhaka. In *Vasishtha Samhita* it is said: "When after giving up inhalation and exhalation, one holds his breath with ease, it is absolute kumbhaka (kevala)." In this pranayama the breath suddenly stops without pooraka and rechaka. The student can retain his breath as long as he likes through this kumbhaka. He attains the state of raja yoga. Through kevala kumbhaka, the knowledge of kundalini arises. Kundalini is aroused and the sushumna is freed from all sorts of obstacles. He attains perfection in hatha yoga.

He who knows pranayama and kevala is the real yogi. What can he not accomplish in the three worlds, who has acquired success in this kevala kumbhaka? Glory, glory to such exalted souls. This kumbhaka cures all diseases and promotes longevity.

What happens to one's consciousness during kevala kumbhaka?

Swami Satyananda: There are three types of kumbhaka. *Kumbhaka* is when the breath stops. *Antaranga kumbhaka* is stopping the breath within, inside the lungs. *Bahiranga kumbhaka* is emptying the lungs and then stopping the breath. These two kumbhakas are well known to most practitioners. But there is a third sort of khumbaka, it is called *kevala kumbhaka*; it is not forced.

When one is doing meditations or practising pranayama, suddenly the mind may become tranquil – it attains equipoise and stops oscillating. At that time the breath stops for a moment. It neither goes in nor out. That is called kevala kumbhaka. But it is only for a short time. When one concentrates in *bhrumadhya*, between the two eyebrows, then *prakash*, the light becomes visible. When the light becomes visible the breath stops. It may only be experienced for a second or two or three, but by gradual practise the concentration on the light in bhrumadhya can be done for two, three, four, five or ten days.

One loses one's grip on time, space and object. The grip of self-awareness is lost, and the breath spontaneously suspends. During that time, the consciousness hangs in between, neither in the body nor beyond; the self hangs as if in suspension between the body and the higher self. This is a difficult matter for people to understand. The poet saints of India – Kabir, Nanak and Surdas, have all written poems on this phenomena. If one reads and tries to understand the everyday songs and poems by Mirabai, by Kabir, and by many others, this state of kevala kumbhaka is considered to be very important. In fact, the sadhu or the yogi who performs underground samadhi, *bhu samadhi*, is using this same system.

Of course, people used to consider them bogus, but now science is testing yogis who take underground samadhi by remote control systems. Their radial pulses are checked, their cardiac behaviour, their metabolic systems, their skin resistances, their blood flow – everything is checked by remote control systems. This has shown that it is not bogus. There are many yogis who have failed. They have died. This is also true.

In which part of the pranic body is kevala kumbhaka experienced?

Swami Satyananda: There are innumerable varieties of kumbhakas described in the hatha yogic tradition, but none can equal the kevala kumbhaka, because in no other kumbhaka does the prana become steady. This is described by Adi Shankaracharya in *Yoga Taravali* (v. 8–10):

Bandhatrayaabhyaasavipaaka jaataam
Vivarjitaam rechaka poorakaabhyaam.
Visheshayantee vishayapravaaham
Vidyaam bhaje kevalakumbharoopam.

Anaahate chetasi saavadhaanaih
Abhyaasashoorairanubhooyamaanaa.
Samstambhita shvaasamanah prachaaraa
Saa jrimbhate kevala kumbhakashreeh.

Sahasrashah santu hatheshu kumbhaah
Sambhaavyate kevala kumbha eva.
Kumbhottame yatra tu rechapoorau
Praanasya na praakritavaikritaakhyau.

Gradually, through the mastery of the three bandhas, exhalation and inhalation are suspended, and a detachment towards undesirable objects arises. I bow to this vidya, known as kevala khumbaka. (8)

When a person focuses his mind gradually on anahata, and practices (the three bandhas) with courage, then slowly he experiences the precious state of kevala khumbaka. (9)

The school of hatha yoga talks about thousands of kinds of pranayama. Among them, kevala khumbaka is the most respected. In this state of kevala khumbaka, there is no movement of breath outward or inward. (10)

How does kumbhaka culminate in samadhi?

Swami Satyananda: The Sanskrit word kevala means 'only', and kumbhaka means 'breath retention' or 'cessation'. The word *kevala* is directly connected with the word *kaivalya* meaning 'onlyness', but is another name for *samadhi*, *nirvana* or supreme enlightenment and union. Therefore kevala and kaivalya mean that experience which is beyond duality, beyond mere conception, beyond words. Any description of the experience immediately distorts it and can never adequately convey its essence. For this reason, the words kevala and kaivalya are used as a suitable nondescription of the indescribable. In *Hatha Yoga Pradipika* (4:51–52) it is said:

Baahyavaayuryathaa leenastatha madhyo na samshayah;
Svasthaane sthirataameti pavano manasaa saha.

Evamabhyasamaanasya vaayumaarge divaanisham;
Abhyaasaajjeeryate vaayurmanastatraiva leeyate.

When the external breath is suspended, likewise the middle one (i.e. shakti in sushumna is suspended). Without a doubt, prana and mind become still in their own place (i.e. brahmarandhra). (51)

Verily, practising with the breath (prana) day and night through the course of prana (sushumna), prana and mind become absorbed there. (52)

Kevala kumbhaka is the spontaneous cessation of breath that occurs with the state of samadhi, attained through pranayama and the meditation methods of raja yoga. If kevala kumbhaka arises, then samadhi must also simultaneously occur. One goes with the other.

What is kevali pranayama?

Swami Niranjanananda: Kevali pranayama is in fact ajapa japa. As long as a human being is alive, one keeps on repeating the ajapa mantra with each breath. Often the attention is diverted and awareness of the mantra is lost, yet the process continues spontaneously. This state is called *kevali*. When awareness of the mantra is added, it becomes *ajapa japa*. In *Gheranda Samhita* (5:86) this is described:

Hankaarena bahiryaati sahkaarena vishetpunah;
Shatshataani divaaraatrau sahasraanyekavimshatih;
Ajapaam naama gaayatreem jeevo japati sarvadaa.

The soul of every living being repeats *Ham* with each exhalation and *So* with each inhalation. Every human being takes 21,600 breaths during one day and night. This is called (*Hamso* or *Soham*) ajapa gayatri. Every living being always keeps on repeating this mantra.

Sage Gheranda makes a differentiation between the conscious practice and the spontaneous mantra of the breath which goes on automatically. In his opinion, a person's only duty, therefore, is to practise kevali. During ajapa japa the breath is imagined in three main centres of the body. When inhaling, the breath is felt rising up from mooladhara and reaching *nasikagra*, the nosetip, after crossing anahata chakra. When exhaling, the presence of the breath is felt moving downward from the nosetip to mooladhara. As the breath crosses the centres step by step, the mind is focused there. This is described in *Gheranda Samhita* (5:87):

Moolaadhaare yathaa hamsastathaa hi hridi pankaje;
Tathaa naasaaputadvandve tribhirhamsasamaagamah.

The air goes in and out through three places: mooladhara, the heart lotus, and the two nostrils.

How can kevali pranayama be practised in daily life?
Swami Niranjanananda: In the initial stages practising awareness of the mantra and of one's own internal state is maintained. This can prove helpful in self-analysis or introspection. During the day when one is busy with work, contact with the internal personality is lost and many perplexities are faced due to being involved in the vicious circles of the mind. In this externalized state one often wants to selfishly fulfil one's own wishes and desires. Consequently, in order to get to know the state of the mind and to maintain awareness, one should practise (*Hamso* or *Soham*) ajapa regularly each day.

Gheranda Samhita (5:92–93) describes the advanced practice:

Yaavajjeevam japenmantramajapaasankhyakevalam;
Adyaavadhi dhritam sankhyaavibhramam kevalee krite.

Ata eva hi kartavyah kevaleekumbhako naraih;
Kevalee chaajapaasankhyaa dvigunaa cha manonmanee.

Throughout life living beings spontaneously keep on repeating the ajapa mantra, yogis must do it consciously. (92)

241

In kevali kumbhaka there is no regular respiration. (If the rate of reduction of respiration) is doubled, then manonmani (extreme bliss) takes place. (93)

For the advanced practitioners that are being addressed in these sutras, extended periods of practice are possible throughout the day, but this is not possible for busy commuters with multiple responsibilities. Also, advanced practitioners would have gradually adapted to the effects of prolonged kumbhaka by perfecting previous pranayamas (such as moorcha kumbhaka) in terms of the nervous system, metabolism, lifestyle, attitudes, etc.

How often should ajapa japa with breath retention be practised?

Swami Niranjanananda: For the normal practitioner today, ajapa japa should be practised once or twice a day. Sage Gheranda teaches that this practice must be done at least three times a day and recommends the three *sandhyas*, times of confluence of energies, at sunrise, noon and sunset. In *Gheranda Samhita* (5:94–96) it is written:

Naasaabhyaam vaayumaakrishya kevalam kumbhakam charet;
Ekaadikachatuhshashtim dhaarayetprathame dine.

Kevaleemashtadhaa kuryaadyaame yaame dine dine;
Atha vaa panchadhaa kuryaadyathaa tatkathayaami te.

Praatarmadhyaahnasaayaahne madhyaraatre chaturthake;
Trisandhyamatha vaa kuryaatsamamaane dine dine.

Drawing the air through the nostrils, just spontaneously suspend the breath, performing this breath retention known as kevali up to 64 times on the first day. (94)

Kevali kumbhaka should be practised daily eight times (once every three hours) or practised five times as I specify: in the early morning, noon, twilight, midnight and in the fourth quarter of the night. Or practised three times at the three sandhyas (at sunrise, noon and at sunset). (95–96)

What is the culmination of pranayama?

Swami Niranjanananda: In concluding his chapter on pranayama, Sage Gheranda says that for those who achieve perfection in kevali pranayama, self-knowledge and knowledge of the science of yoga dawn, and nothing is impossible in this world. This is written in *Gheranda Samhita* (5:97–98):

Panchavaaram dine vriddhirvaaraikam cha dine tathaa;
Ajapaaparimaanam cha yaavatsiddhih prajaayate.

Praanaayaamam kevaleem cha tadaa vadati yogavit;
Kevaleekumbhake siddhe kim na sidhyati bhootale.

Until this practice is perfected, keep on increasing the scale by five times along with ajapa gayatri. (97)

One who perfects pranayama and kevali is called a real knower of yoga. Having mastered kevali kumbhaka, what cannot be achieved in this world? (98)

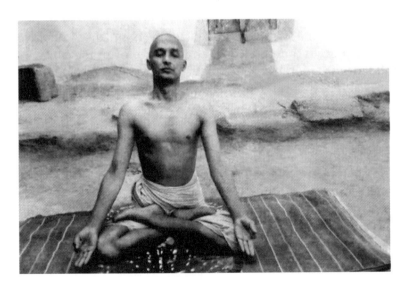

243

10

Pranayama in Spiritual Life

PRANAYAMA AND THE SOUL

What is meant by purification through pranayama?

Swami Sivananda: Tamas and rajas constitute the covering or veil. This veil is removed by the practice of pranayama. After the veil is removed, the real nature of the soul is realized. The chitta by itself is made up of sattwic particles, but it is enveloped by rajas and tamas, just as the fire is enveloped by smoke. There is no purificatory action greater than pranayama. Pranayama gives purity, and the light of knowledge shines.

The karma of the yogi, which covers up discriminative knowledge, is annihilated by the practice of pranayama. By the magic panorama of desire, the essence, which is luminous by nature, is covered up and the *jiva* or individual soul is directed towards vice. This karma of the yogi which covers up the light and binds him to repeated births, is reduced by the practice of pranayama, and is eventually destroyed. After this veil of the light has been removed, the mind can easily concentrate. It will be quite steady, like the flame in a windless place, as the disturbing energy has been removed.

When the prana vayu moves in akasha tattwa, the breathing becomes less, and at this time it is easy to stop the breath. The velocity of the mind is slowly lessened by the pranayama. Vairagya arises.

Why is pranayama important in spiritual life?

Swami Satyananda: Pranayama practices establish a healthy body by removing blockages in the pranamaya kosha, enabling increased absorption and retention of prana. The spiritual seeker requires tranquillity of mind as an essential prelude to spiritual practice.

To this end, many pranayama techniques use *kumbhaka*, breath retention, to establish control over the flow of prana, calming the mind and controlling the thought process.

Once the mind has been stilled and prana flows freely in the nadis and chakras, the doorway to the evolution of consciousness opens, leading the aspirant into higher dimensions of spiritual experience.

What are the outcomes and signs that the nadis have been purified by pranayama?

Swami Sivananda: If the breath is unsteady, the mind is unsteady. If the breath is steady and calm, the mind is steady and calm. A yogi attains longevity by the practice of pranayama. Therefore, the practice of pranayama is indispensable.

The fundamental aim of pranayama is to unite the prana and the apana, and to take the united prana-apana slowly up towards the crown of the head. The fruit of pranayama is the awakening of the sleeping kundalini shakti.

By the practice of pranayama one can become a veritable God. Certain symptoms manifest when the nadis are purified. One's body becomes light and slender. A peculiar lustre comes into the eyes, and a remarkable glow into the countenance. The voice becomes sweet and melodious. The breath can be retained for a long time. The anahata sounds can be heard emanating quite audibly from the heart lotus. The digestive fire is augmented, perfect health is enjoyed, and one is cheerful and happy. In *Hatharatnavali* (3:98) it is written:

Praanaayaama paro yogee so'pi vishnu maheshvarah;
Sarvadevamayo yogee tasyaavajnaam na kaarayet.

One who has mastered pranayama is like Vishnu and Maheshwara. The yogi is like all the gods. Therefore, he should never be disobeyed.

PRANAYAMA AND MEDITATION

Does the perfection of pranayama spontaneously lead to the state of meditation?

Swami Satyananda: When pranayama is mastered, one automatically enters into a state called meditation or concentration. This state can be attained by other methods as well, but pranayama is a scientific basis for clearing the consciousness of all the obstructions that lie before it. Therefore, the practice of pranayama has to be done intelligently and patiently. Pranayama must be seen in relation to the awakening of yoga. In the *Yoga Chudamani Upanishad* (v. 108) it is written:

Praanaayaamo bhavedevam paatakendhanapaavakaha;
Bhavodadhimahaasetuh prochyate yogibhih sadaa.

In this way, pranayama becomes fire for the fuel of sin, and has always been regarded by the yogis as a great bridge for crossing the ocean of the world.

How does pranayama fit into the sequence of yogic practices?

Swami Niranjanananda: Pranayama is not a stand-alone yogic practice. In the ashtanga yoga of Sage Patanjali's *Yoga Sutras*, it is preceded by sustained practice of yamas, niyamas and asanas, and is followed by pratyahara, dharana, dhyana and samadhi. A balanced, sequential movement from gross to subtle, from annamaya kosha to anandamaya kosha, is the aim. In *Hatha Yoga Pradipika* (1:67) it has been said:

Peethaani kumbhakaashchitraa divyaani karanaani cha;
Sarvaanyapi hathaabhyaase raajayogaphalaavadhih.

Asanas, various types of kumbhaka (pranayama) and the other various means of illumination should all be practised in the hatha yoga system until success in raja yoga is attained.

In this context, the aim of pranayama is to perfect pratyahara. In the traditional texts *pratyahara* has been described not just as sense withdrawal, but as the state where every sensory input is perceived as a manifestation of the Supreme, and in which the pranic capacity is expanded to the extent that the breath can be retained for three hours. The *Shiva Samhita* (3:57) states:

> *Yaamamaatram yadaa dharttum samarthah syaattadaadbhutah;*
> *Pratyaahaarastadaiva syaannaamtaraa bhavati dhru vam.*

> When one attains the power of holding the breath for three hours, then certainly the wonderful state of pratyahara is reached without fail.

How does pranayama help prepare one for meditation?

Swami Satyananda: The pranayama breathing techniques influence the brain. The brain has two hemispheres which are connected with the two nostrils. The breath inhaled through the left nostril influences the right hemisphere and the breath inhaled through the right nostril influences the left hemisphere. The two hemispheres of the brain and the two breathing systems are related to the sympathetic and parasympathetic nervous systems.

The right nostril corresponds with the life force. The left nostril represents and corresponds with the mental force. If one meditates when the left nostril is flowing there will be a lot of visions, psychic visions, forms, and imaginations, but no meditation. If one tries to meditate when the right nostril is flowing, it will not be possible either, as the mind will be too active or hyperactive. Therefore, those who want to meditate must know that the right time for meditation is when both nostrils are flowing equally. When pranayama is practised, both hemispheres of the brain are influenced, creating balance between the sympathetic and parasympathetic nervous systems. At that time, one should go ahead with meditation. When there is harmony in the nervous system and when there is harmony in the brain, the mind separates itself from the senses.

How does controlling the prana prepare the mind for meditation?

Swami Satyananda: Pranayama is an essential prelude to and integral part of, kriya yoga and various other meditation practices. Control of one's breath leads to control of prana. In turn, control of prana implies control of one's mind. By regulating the flow of prana in the body one can tranquillize the mind and free it, at least for some time, of the incessant conflicts and thoughts that make higher awareness difficult. By manipulating prana in the psychic body one is able to make the mind a suitable vessel for meditative experience. The mind and prana are directly related. If the mind is like a restless monkey jumping from one thought to another, how can meditation be successfully practised? The aim of both pranayama and meditation techniques is the same: perfect receptivity and quiescence of mind so that one can know higher experience.

Pranayama is an indispensable tool. Meditation can be experienced without pranayama, but pranayama is the supercharger that makes meditation possible for most people. Ramana Maharshi spoke of this when he said, "The principle underlying the system of yoga is that the source of thought on the one hand, and of breath and vital forces on the other, is one and the same. In other words, the breath, vital forces, the physical body, and even the mind are all no more than forms of prana or energy. Therefore, if any of them are effectively controlled then the other is automatically brought under control."

Why does pranayama come before pratyahara in Sage Patanjali's ashtanga yoga?

Swami Niranjanananda: In the ashtanga yoga of Sage Patanjali, there is asana, pranayama and then pratyahara. Why does pranayama come before pratyahara? What is the purpose of pranayama and how is it practised? According to Sri Krishna, one should practise shutting out all thought of external enjoyments, with the gaze fixed on the space between the eyebrows, and regulate the prana shakti. Then regulate the prana and the apana which flow as breath within the nostrils. Only after regulating the prana is it possible to bring the senses, mind and intellect under control. Sri Krishna states in the *Bhagavad Gita* (5:27–28):

Sparshaankritvaa bahirbaahyaamshchakshushchaivaantare bhruvoh
Pranaapaanau samau kritvaa naasaabhyantarachaarinau.

Yatendriyamanobuddhirmunirmokshaparaayanah
Vigatechchhaabhayakrodho yah sadaa mukta eva sah.

Shutting out all thoughts of the external environment, with the gaze fixed on the space between the eyebrows, having equalized the currents of prana and apana flowing within the nostrils, controlled the senses, mind and intellect, such a contemplative soul, intent on liberation and free from desire, fear and anger, is truly free forever. (27–28)

These are instructions for meditation. The gaze is fixed at the eyebrow centre with the image of the flame. The mind must have something to hold its attention, otherwise it will waver. The sensation of the coming and going of the breath is experienced, its coolness and warmth, the flows of prana and apana. In this way the senses are shut off and one enters the inner compartment of the mind where the flame is held steady. When pratyahara is extended, one becomes free from desire, fear and anger, and attains liberation.

Our guru, Swami Satyananda, used to tell the story of a bird flying over the ocean. Halfway through its flight, the bird becomes tired. What will it do? It cannot land in the middle of the ocean to rest, so it will try to find a piece of floating wood or maybe some dry land to rest on. If it is unable to find land, it will always return to the same piece of floating wood to rest and then again take off. In yoga one also needs an *adhara*, a support, a foundation, a basis, an object on which to rest, relax, energize and then continue. To perfect pratyahara and achieve *dharana*, inner concentration, pranayama is the support.

How does pranayama help one to attain pratyahara?

Swami Niranjanananda: In the *Bhagavad Gita* Arjuna asks Sri Krishna, "Can you tell me how one can perfect pratyahara?" and Sri Krishna tells Arjuna that one has to practise pranayama. Without the practice of pranayama the energy cannot be awakened within oneself, because right now all the energies are directed outwards. In the *Bhagavad Gita* (3:42) Sri Krishna says to Arjuna:

*Indriyaani paraanyaahuh indriyebhyah param manah
Manasastu paraa buddhiryo buddheh paratastu sah.*

The senses are said to be superior to the body; superior to the senses is the mind; superior to the mind is the intellect; and superior even to the intellect is the atma, the inner spirit.

When one is identified with the senses, one is identified with the lower level of the personality. The higher level of the personality, beyond the senses, is the mind. Realize that. Higher than mind is the intellect, *viveka buddhi*, the discriminative faculty. Realize that. Higher than the discriminative ability is the still and silent nature of the Self, which is the *atma*. If one is to move from the realm of the senses to the realm of the inner spirit, one has to be able to harmonize the body, which is the experiencer

250

of the senses. The body is controlled by prana; the senses are controlled by prana. Therefore, one must practise pranayama.

How does pranayama support the technique of nada yoga?

Swami Satyananda: Pranayama is a practice for intensifying the meditative technique of nada yoga. In the *Yoga Chudamani Upanishad* (v. 115) it is said:

> *Gaganam pavane praapte dhvanirutpadyate mahaan;*
> *Ghantaa adeenaam pravaadyaanaam naadasiddhirudeeritaa.*

> When the prana rises into the sky, inner sounds of musical instruments are produced, like the bell and so on, and the perfection of inner sound is achieved.

Pranayama makes one more sensitive to the inner environment. In this way one is more able to perceive the subtle nada. For this reason, one should aim to practise nada yoga immediately after pranayama practice.

How can higher states of consciousness be attained by practising bhramari?

Swami Niranjanananda: In *Gheranda Samhita* nada yoga is discussed along with bhramari. The practical technique of bhramari pranayama is slightly different from the technique used in nada yoga, and is considered as the initial stage to balance the mind and internalize the awareness. It is this simple stage that is taught as a pranayama practice.

The practice of bhramari as nada yoga develops awareness of the subtle inner sounds. These states are described in *Gheranda Samhita* (5:79–84):

> *Ardharaatre gate yogee jantoonaam shabdavarjite;*
> *Karnau pidhaaya hastaabhyaam kuryaatpoorakakumbhakam.*

> *Shrinuyaaddakshine karne naadamantargatam shubham;*
> *Prathamam jhillikaanaadam vamsheenaadam tatah param.*

Meghajharjharabhramaree ghantaa kaasyam tatah param;
Tureebhereemridangaadininaadaanekadundubhih.

Evam naanaavidho naado jaayate nityamabhyasaat;
Anaahatasya shabdasya tasya shabdasya yo dhvanih.

Dhvanerantargatam jyotirjyotirantargatam manah;
Tanmano vilayam yaati tadvishnoh paramam padam;
Evam bhraamareesamsiddhih samaadhisiddhimaapnuyaat.

Japaadashta gunam dhyaanam dhyaanaadashtagunam tapah;
Tapaso'shtagunam gaanam gaanaatparataram nahi.

After midnight, in a quiet place where no sound of any living being is heard, a yogi should practise inhalation and breath retention while closing the ears with the hands. (79)

One listens to internal sounds with the right ear. First the sound of a grasshopper, then the sound of a flute, then the thundering of clouds, then the sound of a cymbal or small drum, then the humming sound of bees, a bell, a big gong, a trumpet, a kettledrum, a mridanga or a drum, a dundubhi, etc., are heard. (80–81)

Thus, by practising daily, one has the experience of listening to various sounds and the sound of the shabda (sacred sound or vibration) is produced in anahata. In its resonance comes the internal vision of the twelve-petalled lotus in the heart. With the merging of the mind into the flame, one attains the lotus feet of Lord Vishnu. Thus by perfecting bhramari kumbhaka, one attains the siddhi of samadhi. (82–83)

Dhyana is eight times superior to japa, tapas (austerity) is eight times superior to dhyana, and music is eight times superior to tapas. There is nothing greater than music. (84)

After practising bhramari, one continues breathing quietly with the ears closed, trying to listen to the sounds produced inside by slowly internalizing the awareness and making it subtle. In the beginning, the sound of the breathing is heard. As one continues with the practice, awareness of a sound will come, and one must try to remain totally aware of that particular sound to the exclusion of all other sounds.

After several days or weeks of regular practice that particular sound will become increasingly clear and distinct. One must keep on listening to that sound with complete awareness, letting the awareness flow only towards that sound and forgetting all other sounds and thoughts. Sensitivity of perception will be further enhanced by continuous practice.

As the practice deepens, the heartbeat is heard. Going deeper still, the sound of the blood flowing through the veins is heard. Going deeper still, speech will be heard, as if someone is speaking inside. Very far away, the sound of grasshoppers, sparrows and music is heard. In this way, gradually, one's perception becomes more and more acute and sensitive.

In this stage, all these sounds are heard while keeping the ears closed. These sounds are produced inside quite naturally. Some sounds are produced from memory, and when the region of memory and chitta is crossed, subtle sounds are heard rather than gross sounds. When subtle sound is also crossed, then only nada is heard, which is called *anahad nada*, unbroken sound.

Nada or sound waves are related to a *jyoti*, a flame or light. Light is linked with the mind. When there is complete union with the mind or nada, the experience of God occurs. So with bhramari, siddhi or mastery of samadhi is achieved.

The sage also says clearly that the significance or importance of music is even greater than *dhyana*, meditation, and *tapas*, austerity. In meditation the mind has a blissful experience, eight times better than that of japa. Austerity gives an experience eight times better again, but in music or nada one experiences bliss eight times better than with tapas. Nothing is greater than nada.

253

Sage Gheranda has mentioned here that sound is related to a flame or light, light is related to mind and mind is related to *nada* or sound. This means a cycle has been created: nada, light, mind and nada (sound). The nada which is being discussed here is *parananda*, transcendental bliss. Slowly, by crossing different states, listening to gross sounds and subtle nada, a subtle state is entered. One listens to subtle sound, experiences it and then enters into parananda.

The state of parananda itself is the state of light or perception. This state of knowledge or perception influences the mind, and when the mind is engulfed by this experience, only nada is heard. Up-down, right-left, in front-behind, everywhere, nothing but nada is heard. In this parananda, God is experienced. This is the ultimate state of bhramari. For this, total patience and effort are essential. If one is firmly determined about the practice, wonderful results will be achieved.

What is experienced when advanced bhramari is practised?

Swami Sivananda: The joy which the practitioner gets in making the kumbhaka is unlimited and indescribable. In the beginning, the heat of the body is increased as the circulation of blood is quickened. In the end the body heat is decreased by perspiration. By success in bhramari kumbhaka, the yogic student attains success in samadhi.

How does pranayama induce dhyana?

Swami Satyananda: Pranayama is the gateway to dhyana. Through pranayama a sadhaka can go as deep as he wants. Nothing has to be done except to go on practising pranayama with jalandhara, uddiyana and moola bandhas, and some of the kriyas. There is no need to control or fight with the mind. Just do the practices for ten or fifteen minutes every day and in the course of time the mind will enter dhyana. This is the hatha yoga system.

PRANAYAMA AND KUNDALINI

How important is purifying the nadis for the ascent of kundalini in sushumna?

Swami Sivananda: *Nadi shuddhi*, or purification of the nadis, is an important matter in the early stage of yoga. If there are impurities in the nadis, the ascent of kundalini in sushumna is seriously retarded. Purity in the nadis facilitates the ascent of kundalini. Pranayama brings about quick purification of the nadis. Nadi shuddhi is the basis of yoga. It is the foundation of yoga. It is the first part of yoga.

What part does pranayama play in awakening the kundalini?

Swami Satyananda: The greatest objective that pranayama has to fulfil is to awaken the kundalini. Awakening of kundalini is a moment of mental crisis when man takes a new birth, enters a new area of experience and is born into a new area of existence. For pranayama sadhana, all the practices of hatha yoga must be done. If one wants transcendental experience, many rules and regulations must be observed for successful, effective pranayama. Through the practice of pranayama, along with spiritual awakening or the awakening of kundalini, a very great part is played in the evolution of the general intelligence of humanity.

Why is pranayama important in the awakening of kundalini shakti?

Swami Satyananda: The rishis and munis did not design pranayama for the sake of supplying extra oxygen to the body. It is one of the most powerful tools available for the awakening of sushumna nadi or kundalini shakti.

There are thousands of billions of cells in the brain which live in a chaotic way, without any discipline or unity. This is shown as random brainwave activity when measured on an EEG machine. How are they to be blended together as one pulsating unit? These cells are very important because they are the jumping forms of energy, *shakti*. They are the bindu shakti, om shakti, manas shakti, and chitta shakti. They comprise the totality of a person's brainwave activity.

When the basic elements of a person's brain are moving in a chaotic fashion so will that person's thinking processes. Pranayama has a scheme for it. The chaotic elements of the brain cannot be organized or disciplined or brought to order without first awakening the kundalini. The brain is controlled by the chakras and nadis. The three most important nadis are ida, pingala and sushumna. Unless a balance is created between ida and pingala nadis through the practices of hatha yoga, including pranayama, it is not possible to create a balance within the mind. The practices of pranayama are of major importance because they help to first purify and balance the flows of ida and pingala nadis, which awakens sushumna nadi and kundalini.

What is the most direct way of awakening sushumna?
Swami Niranjanananda: When the two forces of ida and pingala become active, the third channel of sushumna becomes active. It is a fact that when two opposing forces are equal and balanced, a third force arises. By bringing positive and negative currents together, machinery can be operated. Similarly, when the body and mind are united, a third force arises. This force is called *sushumna*, the spiritual energy. Ida is the negative charge, pingala is the positive charge and sushumna is the neutral. While *ida* and *pingala* conduct mental and physical energy, sushumna conducts a higher form of cosmic energy. The pranic and mental energies are finite whereas the energy of sushumna is infinite.

When sushumna is active, the breath flows through both nostrils simultaneously. Normally this happens for a few minutes when the breath dominance changes over from one nostril to the other, which usually takes place every ninety minutes. Sushumna flows after practising pranayama, prayer and meditation. When sushumna flows, the whole brain operates, but only half the brain is active during the flow of ida or pingala. At the time of sushumna, both *karmendriyas* and *jnanendriyas*, physical organs and mental organs, function simultaneously and the person becomes very powerful. Feelings of equanimity and steadiness arise, because sushumna is the conductor of *mahaprana*, the kundalini energy. Meditative states dawn spontaneously, even in the middle of a traffic jam. The flow of sushumna is considered to be the most favourable for any type of sadhana. Sushumna represents the integration and harmony of opposites at all levels.

Human evolution depends on the awakening of prana shakti, as much as it depends on optimum health of the body. All yogic practices purify the pranas, but pranayama is considered the principal among these. The awakening of prana takes place when the nadis flow regularly, rhythmically and continuously and no blockages or physiological discomfort are encountered in the breathing process. This stage is known as *pranotthana*, awakening of the pranas, more specifically of ida and pingala. When the awakening of ida and pingala occurs, sushumna awakens. The awakening of this third force is considered the most important event in pranayama, kriya yoga and kundalini yoga. Pranayama actually begins with the awakening of sushumna, because then the pranic field expands.

Why is a regulated lifestyle important for advanced pranayama practice?
Swami Satyananda: For the awakening of kundalini, it is important that sushumna nadi be purified. In order to purify sushumna, one must practise a lot of pranayama. When a lot of pranayama is practised, one must take care of many details in life. The rules and regulations which control the practices of prana in relation to food and life must be known and adhered to. This is a form of spiritual discipline, and the person who follows it will never feel any difficulty, nor any sense of punishment or restriction, because the practice of pranayama is necessary to awaken sushumna.

The practice of pranayama means practising kumbhaka. Kumbhaka is the ultimate definition of pranayama. In conjunction with pranayama, the bandhas must be practised. When the bandhas are performed, the mental and psychic systems are affected. If one's stomach, mind, or emotions are constipated, or if one's family or social life is too complicated, or if a person's mental personality lives like a vagabond dog, just imagine what the practice of pranayama with bandhas is going to do!

Strong kumbhaka with jalandhara, uddiyana and moola bandha creates heat in the body. This heat is known as the fire of yoga. It is not only spiritual or psychic in nature, it is also physical and affects the metabolism as well as the psycho-spiritual system. When enough heat is created, there is a powerful explosion and an awakening takes place. How is one to maintain balance in the heat that has been created by the awakening? For this, there are special rules and regulations given in the yogic texts, which say, "Neither too much eating, nor too much fasting; neither too much sleeping, nor too much vigil; neither too much talking, nor too much silence." In *Hatha Yoga Pradipika* (1:15) it is written:

Atyaahaarah prayaasashva prajalpo niyamagrahah;
Janasangashcha laulyam cha shadbhiryogo vinashyati.

Overeating, exertion, talkativeness, adhering to rules, being in the company of common people and unsteadiness (wavering mind) are the six (causes) which destroy yoga.

Extremes are far from helpful on the path of awakening. The practitioner has to understand the important things: proper food, adequate sleep, and the right kind of social interaction. Although Yogi Swatmarama advised that a sadhaka should not adhere to strict rules and regulations, the guru's instructions must be followed. As far as social rituals and religious doctrines are concerned, it is unnecessary that they be maintained for spiritual progress. Sadhana is not

258

dependent on social morals nor are its effects promoted by religious practices. Adhering to rules makes one 'narrow-minded'. Yoga is meant to expand the consciousness, not to limit it. All these things create a balance, and they also balance the complications that could arise due to the awakening.

What role do the various pranayama techniques have in awakening kundalini?

Swami Satyananda: The present amount of pranic energy is insufficient to activate silent areas of the brain. The prime objective of pranayama is to create a greater quantum of prana, change the nature of the electrical forces within the pranic body, and then transmit it to the silent areas. When pranayama has been mastered, prana can be transferred to any part of the body. Pranayama increases vitality and ensures good health, but it is more than just a breathing exercise – it is intended to disturb the sleeping kundalini. In *Hatha Yoga Pradipika* (2:41) it says:

Vidhivatpraanasamyaamairnaadeechakre vishodhite;
Sushumnaavadanam bhittvaa sukhaadvishati maarutah.

By systematically restraining the prana (breath), the nadis and chakras are purified. Thus the prana bursts open the doorway to sushumna and easily enters it.

The different forms of pranayama prepare the channels or media through which the energy must flow. Not all pranayamas are specifically intended to awaken kundalini. Certain pranayamas are practised to purify the carrying channels, the *nadis*. Some are intended to create heat in the system while others stimulate ajna chakra to function as a monitor. For example, there is an important pranayama known as ujjayi which clears pingala for the ascension of prana.

The whole science of pranayama is based on retention of prana known as kumbhaka. Inhalation and exhalation are incidental. Kumbhaka means pranayama and pranayama means kumbhaka. Those aspirants who are keen and working on this new project of awakening the silent areas of the brain should prepare themselves slowly by perfecting kumbhaka. Scientific studies on pranayama have shown that during kumbhaka an increased supply of blood is poured into the brain and at the same time extra heat is generated within the system.

How can pranayama influence human evolution?

Swami Satyananda: Pranayama does not have as much to do with the lungs and the heart as it has to do with the brain. It is primarily an exercise of the lobes of the brain rather than an exercise for the lungs and heart. When pranayama is practised, the lungs receive some extra fresh air and it affects the rhythm of the heart; primarily, however, pranayama is directly to do with the brain.

When one breathes in through the left nostril, the right side of the brain is activated. When one inhales through the right nostril, the left half of the brain is activated. The breath in the left nostril has a slightly lower temperature than the breath which flows through the right one. This is why in yoga the left nostril is known as *chandra swara*, meaning the moon, which is cool, and the right one is known as *surya swara*, meaning the sun, which is warm or hot. The effect on the brain is the same, cooling and heating. So, pranayama is essentially an exercise of the brain. Just as one exercises to improve the biceps and triceps in the body, in the same way pranayama is done to exercise the brain.

In pranayama, the breath is retained, it is stopped for one second, two, ten or thirty. When the breath is retained, impulses are directed downwards through the spine to the perineum. The perineum is the area between the excretory and urinary organs. In yoga it is known as *sukra nadi*. In sukra nadi there is a gland, a tiny gland and this gland is considered to be very important in relation to man's future evolution. Many scholars have written about this. If books on kundalini yoga by the great scholars of the East and

West are read, one comes to understand that this kundalini has something to do with the coming evolutionary cycle of humanity.

Humanity has evolved from instinct to intellect, and now from intellect mankind is going to evolve further. With the awakening of that kundalini, another evolutionary cycle is stepped into. This is the inevitable destiny of man. It cannot be escaped. It has to be. The mind which exists today, and the consciousness which will exist in 5,000 years, cannot be the same. A different type of consciousness, a different kind of thinking, will come to humanity. When pranayama is practised, awakening takes place. And with that awakening transformation in the quality of the mind and transformation in the quality of personality takes place.

PERFECTION

Do higher qualities arise from the practice of pranayama?
Swami Niranjanananda: Pranayama initiates a process in the physical body whereby the energy molecules and the mental forces which interact with one another in life and consciousness, are transformed. When the molecules of mind are transformed, higher qualities such as love, compassion and unity arise.

Matter is energy and, therefore, the physical body can be transformed into energy. The body is rendered extremely subtle and pure through the process of yoga, and accordingly transformed. Pranayama is a key method. When the yogic texts state that through pranayama one can control one's circumstances and character, and harmonize the individual life with the cosmic life, they are referring to the power of pranayama to bring about such an intrinsic transformation.

How does perfection of hatha yoga through pranayama lead to raja yoga?
Swami Sivananda: In *Vasishtha Samhita* it says, "when after giving up inhalation and exhalation, one holds his

261

breath with ease, it is absolute kumbhaka (kevala)." In this pranayama the breath is suddenly stopped without pooraka and rechaka. The student can retain his breath as long as he likes through this kumbhaka. He attains the state of raja yoga.

Through this kevala kumbhaka the knowledge of kundalini arises. Kundalini is aroused and the sushumna is freed from all sorts of obstacles. The sadhaka attains perfection in hatha yoga. This kumbhaka can be practised three times a day.

He who knows pranayama and kevala is the real yogi. What can he not accomplish in the three worlds, who has acquired success in this kevala kumbhaka? Glory, glory to such exalted souls! This kumbhaka cures all diseases and promotes longevity. In *Shiva Samhita* (3:49–51) it is written:

Poorvaarjitaani karmaani praanaayaamena nishchitam;
Naashayetsaadhako dheemaanihalokodbhavaani cha.

Poorvaajitaani paapaani punyaani vividhaani cha;
Naashayetshodashapraanaayaamena yogi pungavah.

Paapatoolachayaanaahopradahetpralayaagninaa;
Tatah paapavinirmuktah pashchaatpunyaani naashayet.

The wise practitioner surely destroys all his karma, whether acquired in this life or in the past, through the regulation of the breath. (49)

The great yogi destroys by sixteen pranayamas the various virtues and vices accumulated in his past life. (50)

This pranayama destroys sin, as fire burns away a heap of cotton; it makes the yogi free from sin; next it destroys the bonds of all his good actions. (51)

How can pranayama be used as a pathway to samadhi?
Swami Satyananda: In the state of samadhi the prana ceases to flow in the body. Pranayama, therefore, tries to bring about samadhi by directly controlling and eventually stopping

the flow of prana. This leads directly to samadhi. In the monumental yogic scripture called the *Yoga Vasishtha* it says:

> Through these practices (pranayama and meditative practices), the prana can be controlled. In this manner one is freed from sorrow, filled with divine ecstasy and becomes enraptured with the supreme experience. If the prana is controlled, the mind will also become very calm. There is an intimate connection between the mind and prana. If the mind is rendered perfectly quiet, then only Brahman (the Supreme) remains.

What siddhis does perfection in pranayama bestow?

Swami Sivananda: Perfection in pranayama gives the eight major siddhis, namely, anima, mahima, laghima, garima, prapti, prakamya, vashitva, and ishitva.

Anima is the power to make oneself minute, whereas with *mahima* one can become as large as one wants. *Laghima* is the power to make the body as light as a feather and fly thousands of miles through the sky in a minute. With *garima* the body can be made as heavy as a mountain.

By the power of *prapti*, all future events can be predicted, unknown languages can be understood, any disease can be cured, distant sounds can be heard, distant objects can be seen, mystical fragrant odours can be smelled, the sun and the moon can be touched with the tip of one's finger while standing on the Earth, and the language of birds and beasts can be understood. Indeed, all desired objects can be attained.

With *prakamya*, the old skin can be cast off and a youthful appearance assumed for an unusual length of time. One can also enter the body of another person. Adi Shankacharya had this power. He entered the body of the Raja of Benares. Yayati, Tirumulanar and Raja Vikramaditya also had this power.

Vashitva is the power to tame wild beasts and bring them under control. With this power one can make anybody obey one's orders and wishes. The elements can be controlled and one is a master of passions and emotions.

Ishitva is the attainment of all divine powers. This makes one the Lord of the universe. Life can even be given to a dead man. Kabir Das, Tulsidas, Akalkot Swami and many others had this power. If one can control the prana, one can completely control all the forces of the universe, mental and physical. By possessing this power, all the secrets of nature can be penetrated, the events of the past, present and future are known, and such a person becomes one with the Supreme Soul.

In *Shiva Samhita* (3:52) it is written:

Praanaayaamena yogeendro labdhaishvaryaashtakaani vai;
Paapapunyodadhim teertvaa trailokyacharataamiyaat.

The mighty yogi, having attained, through pranayama, the eight sorts of psychic powers, and having crossed the ocean of virtue and vice, moves about freely through the three worlds.

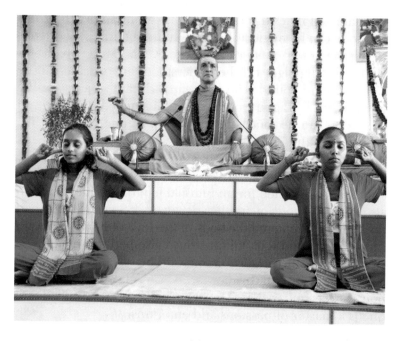

Appendices

Appendix A

Index of Questions

1. Understanding Pranayama

4. Pranayama Sadhana

GENERAL GUIDELINES

PLACE OF PRACTICE

5. Preliminary Breathing Practices

THE SUBTLE BREATH

6. Nadi Shodhana: Purification of the Nadis

ABOUT NADI SHODHANA

GUIDELINES FOR PRACTICE

NADI SHODHANA SADHANA

7. Tranquillizing Pranayamas

8. Vitalizing Pranayamas

ABOUT VITALIZING PRANAYAMAS

SWANA PRANAYAMA: THE PANTING BREATH

BHASTRIKA PRANAYAMA: THE BELLOWS BREATH

9. Advanced Pranayamas

10. Pranayama in Spiritual Life

PRANAYAMA AND THE SOUL

PRANAYAMA AND MEDITATION

PRANAYAMA AND KUNDALINI

Index of Scriptural Quotes

3. Benefits and Effects

6. Nadi Shodhana: Purification of the Nadis

10. Pranayama in Spiritual Life

GHERANDA SAMHITA OF SAGE GHERANDA

1. Understanding Pranayama

3. Benefits and Effects of Pranayama

(5:1) Now I shall explain the technique of pranayama, by the mere practice of which a human being becomes like a deva or god. 62

(5:57) Through the practice of pranayama, travel in space, elimination of diseases and awakening of kundalini is achieved. Bliss manifests in the mind through pranayama and one becomes happy. 83

4. Pranayama Sadhana

(5:2) First select the place and time, eat moderately and purify the nadis. After this, pranayama should be practised. 91

(5:3–7) Yogic practices should not be done in a far-off place, in a forest, in a capital city or in a crowd, otherwise there will be loss of siddhi, lack of success. Far-off places are forbidden because no one can be believed in a distant country, a forest is an insecure place, and in a capital city there is excessive population. Therefore, all three places are prohibited for pranayama. It should be done in a beautiful spiritual region, where food is readily available, and the country is free from internal or external disturbances. Making a hut there, construct a boundary around it. There should be a well or a water source. The ground on which that hut is constructed should be neither too high nor too low, plastered with cow dung, free from insects and in a secluded place. Pranayama should be practised there. 98

(5:8) Yogic practices should not be commenced during winter, extreme cold, summer or the rainy season. If yogic practices are undertaken during these seasons, it leads to the spread of diseases. 101

(5:9) It is correct to start the practices during spring and autumn. When yogic practices are undertaken during these seasons, one certainly attains success and becomes free from diseases. 101

(5:15) It has been said that one attains success by commencing yogic practices during spring and autumn. 102

(5:16) A practitioner who undertakes yoga without moderating the diet suffers from many diseases and does not make progress in yoga. 113

(5:21) The stomach should be half-filled with pleasing, pure, sweet, cooling, oily or lubricating materials until satisfied, and half of the stomach should be left empty. Learned people have termed it mitahara, meaning balance, control or moderation in eating. 113

(5:22) Half of the stomach should be filled with food, a quarter with water and the fourth quarter left empty for the circulation of air. 114

(5:23–25) When commencing yogic practice, one should avoid bitter, sour or acidic, salty and astringent foods, fried food, curd, buttermilk, heavy vegetables, wine, palm nuts and overripe jack fruit. Consuming foods such as horse gram and lentils, pandu fruit, pumpkin and vegetable stems, gourds, berries, limes, garlic, asafoetida, etc., are prohibited. 114

(5:26–27) A beginner should avoid excess travelling, the company of women, or warming himself by the fire. Fresh butter, clarified butter, milk, jaggery, sugar, amalaki, pomegranate, grapes, ripe bananas, etc., should also not be used. 114

(5:28) Cardamom, cloves, nutmeg, stimulants, haritaki and dates can be taken. 115

(5:29) Only foods which are easily digestible, agreeable, lubricating, strengthening and acceptable to the mind should be eaten. Hard, polluted, stale, heating, extremely cold and extremely hot foods should be avoided. 115

(5:30) Early morning bathing and fasting, which cause discomfort to the body, should be discarded. Having only one meal a day, not eating at all or eating between meals should be discontinued. 115

(5:31) Prior to commencing pranayama practice, one should have milk and ghee daily and eat two meals a day, one at noon and one in the evening. 116

(5:9) It is correct to start the practices during spring and autumn. When yogic practices are undertaken during these seasons, one certainly attains success and becomes free from diseases. 129

6. Nadi Shodhana: Purification of the Nadis

(5:34) Sage Gheranda replied: If air cannot flow through the nadis because they are full of waste products, how can pranayama be perfected, and how can tattwa jnana (subtle knowledge) manifest? 141

(5:38–39) Keeping in mind the vayu bija mantra Yam, inhale through the left nostril (chandra marga), repeating the bija mantra 16 times. In the meditative state one should consider this vayu bija to be the colour of bright smoke. Thus after inhalation through the left nostril, one should perform kumbhaka (holding the breath), repeating the mantra 64 times, and then repeating it 32 times perform exhalation through the right nostril. 155

(5:40–42) Raise the fire element (agni tattwa) from the navel centre and meditate on its light associated with earth. Keeping in mind the *Ram* bija and repeating this mantra 16 times one should inhale through the right nostril (surya nadi), perform kumbhaka while repeating it up to 64 times and then exhale through the left nostril, repeating the mantra 32 times. 155

(5:43) Focus the mind on the image of the moon at the nosetip and repeat the bija manta *Tham* 16 times while inhaling through the left nostril. 155

(5:44) One should retain the breath in sushumna, repeating the bija mantra *Vam* 64 times. One should fix the mind on the flow of nectar from the moon at the tip of the nose and clean all the nadis with it. Then one should exhale through the right nostril by repeating the *Lam* bija mantra 32 times. 156

7. Tranquillizing Pranayamas

(5:74) Fill the abdomen by sucking air through the tongue. Retain the air for a short while with the help of kumbhaka and expel it through both nostrils. 167

(5:75) This beneficial sheetali pranayama should always be practised. By practising it, digestive disorders and kapha-pitta disorders do not manifest. 167

(5:72) This is called ujjayi kumbhaka. With it all works are perfected. Diseases from kapha imbalances, nervous and digestive disorders do not manifest. 171

(5:73) Diseases like ama vata, tuberculosis, respiratory disorders, fever and spleen-related disorders are cured. If ujjayi kumbhaka is perfected, old age and death are also managed. 171

(5:70) Inhaling external air through both the nostrils, suck the internal air through the heart and throat and hold it by means of kumbhaka. 173

(5:71) Then emptying the mouth, apply jalandhara bandha, hold the breath to capacity in a manner which does not cause any obstruction. 173

(5:85) Perform breath retention comfortably. Take the mind away from material things and focus it on the eyebrow centre, merging it with the atman. By perfecting moorchha kumbhaka bliss is certainly attained. 179

8. Vitalizing Pranayamas

(5:76) Breathe in and out forcefully through both nostrils, filling and emptying the abdomen like the bellows of a blacksmith. 186

(5:77–78) Repeat this 20 times then hold the breath. The learned ones have named it bhastrika kumbhaka. It should be repeated thus thrice. By practising it, no disease or disorder takes place and a disease-free state is increased day by day. 186

(1:55) Vatakrama, vyutkrama and sheetkrama are the three types of bhalbhati. Practising them eliminates phlegm and mucus from the body. 198

(1:56) The breath is to be inhaled through ida nadi (the left nostril) and exhaled through pingala nadi (the right nostril). Then the breath is inhaled through surya nadi (the right nostril) and exhaled through chandra nadi (the left nostril). 200

290

(1:57) Inhalation and exhalation should be fast; do not hold it. This technique removes kapha dosha. 200

(5:69) This pranayama, surya bheda, is the destroyer of old age and death. It awakens kundalini and the fire inside the body is activated. O Chanda, I have narrated to you the best pranayama known as surya bheda. 209

9. Advanced Pranayamas

(5:54) Nigarbha pranayama is practised without bija mantras; the left hand moves on the left knee (to keep count) of the pranayama consisting of inhalation, retention and exhalation from one to one hundred. 233

(5:55) The highest pranayama has twenty counts, the medium sixteen and the lowest twelve. Thus pranayama has three wings. 233

(5:56) The lowest gives birth to heat or perspiration; through the middle count trembling of the body (especially the spine) is achieved, and by the highest, the practitioner is lifted up from the earth and travels in space. These three (experiences) should all be considered as symptoms of mastery. 234

(5:86) The soul of every living being repeats *Ham* with each exhalation and *So* with each inhalation. Every human being takes 21,600 breaths during one day and night. This is called (*Hamso* or *Soham*) ajapa gayatri. Every living being always keeps on repeating this mantra. 240

(5:87) The air goes in and out through three places: mooladhara, the heart lotus and the two nostrils. 241

(5:92) Throughout life living beings spontaneously keep on repeating the ajapa mantra, yogis must do it consciously. 241

(5:93) In kevali kumbhaka there is no regular respiration. (If the rate of reduction of respiration) is doubled, then manonmani (extreme bliss) takes place. 242

(5:94) Drawing the air through the nostrils, just spontaneously suspend the breath, performing this breath retention known as kevali up to 64 times on the first day. 242

(5:95–96) Kevali kumbhaka should be practised daily eight times (once every three hours) or practised five times as I specify: in the early morning, noon, twilight, midnight and in the fourth quarter of the night. Or practise three times at the three sandhyas (at sunrise, noon and at sunset). 242

(5:97) Until this practice is perfected, keep on increasing the scale by five times along with ajapa gayatri. 243

(5:98) One who perfects pranayama and kevali is called a real knower of yoga. Having mastered kevali kumbhaka, what cannot be achieved in this world? 243

10. Pranayama in Spiritual Life

(5:79) After midnight, in a quiet place where no sound of any living being is heard, a yogi should practise inhalation and breath retention while closing the ears with the hands. 252

(5:80–81) One listens to internal sounds with the right ear. First the sound of a grasshopper, then the sound of a flute, then the thundering of clouds, then the sound of a cymbal or small drum, then the humming sound of bees, a bell, a big gong, a trumpet, a kettledrum, a mridanga or a drum, a dundubhi, etc., are heard. 252

(5:82–83) Thus, by practising daily, one has the experience of listening to various sounds and the sound of the shabda (sacred sound or vibration) is produced in anahata. In its resonance comes the internal vision of the twelve-petalled lotus in the heart. With the merging of the mind into the flame, one attains the lotus feet of Lord Vishnu. Thus by perfecting bhramari kumbhaka, one attains the siddhi of samadhi. 252

(5:84) Dhyana is eight times superior to japa, tapas (austerity) is eight times superior to dhyana, and music is eight times superior to tapas. There is nothing greater than music. 252

1. Understanding Pranayama

3. Benefits and Effects of Pranayama

4. Pranayama Sadhana

(2:36) By the six karmas (shatkarma) one is freed from excesses of the doshas. Then pranayama is practised and success is achieved without strain. 107

(2:14) In the beginning stages of practice, food consisting of milk and ghee is recommended. Upon being established in the practice such restrictions are not necessary. 118

(2:16) All diseases are eradicated by the proper practice of pranayama; all diseases can arise through improper practice. 120

(2:6) Therefore, pranayama should be done daily with a sattwic state of mind so that the impurities are driven out of sushumna nadi and purification occurs. 122

(3:127) All the pranayama methods are to be done with a concentrated mind. The wise man should not let his mind be involved in the modifications (vrittis). 125

(4:29) Mind is the master of the senses, and the breath is the master of the mind . . . 127

6. Nadi Shodhana: Purification of the Nadis

(2:5) When all the nadis and chakras which are full of impurities are purified, then the yogi is able to retain prana. 142

(2:10) When the prana is inhaled through the left nostril, then it must be exhaled through the other. When it is inhaled through the right, hold it inside and then exhale through the other nostril. The yamini who practises in this way, through the right and left nostrils, alternately purifies all his nadis within three months. 146

7. Tranquillizing Pranayamas

(2:54) By drawing the breath in through the mouth, make a hissing sound, without gaping the mouth, and exhale through the nose. By practising this, one becomes a second Kamadeva (god of love). 163

(2:55) He is adored by the circle of yoginis and becomes the controller of creation and dissolution, being without hunger, thirst, sleep and laziness. 163

(2:56) And the sattwa in the body becomes free from all disturbances. Truly, by the aforementioned method one becomes lord of yogis on this earth. 165

(2:57) The wise inhale air through the tongue and practise kumbhaka as (described) before, then exhale the air through the nostrils. 165

(2:58) This kumbhaka called sheetali cures an enlarged stomach or spleen and other related diseases, fever, excess bile, hunger and thirst, and counteracts poisons. 168

(2:51) Closing the mouth, inhale with control and concentration through ida and pingala, so that the breath is felt from the throat to the heart and produces a sonorous sound. 169

(2:52) Do kumbhaka as before and exhale through ida. This removes phlegm from the throat and stimulates the (digestive) fire. 169

(2:53) This pranayama, called ujjayi, can be done while moving, standing, sitting or walking. It removes dropsy and disorders of the nadis and dhatu. 171

(2:69) At the end of inhalation gradually become fixed on jalandhara bandha, then exhale slowly. This is called the fainting or swooning pranayama as it makes the mind inactive and thus confers pleasure. 177

(2:68) Breathe in quickly, making a reverberating sound like the male black bee, and exhale slowly while softly making the sound of the female black bee. By this yogic practice one becomes lord of the yogis and the mind is absorbed in bliss. 181

8. Vitalizing Pranayamas

(2:66) This (bhastrika) quickly arouses kundalini. It is pleasant and beneficial, and removes obstruction due to excess mucus accumulated at the entrance to brahma nadi. 195

(2:67) This kumbhaka called bhastrika enables the three granthis to be broken. Thus it is the duty of the yogi to practise bhastrika. 195

9. Advanced Pranayamas

HATHARATNAVALI OF SRINIVASA BHATTA MAHAYOGINDRA

(3:96) By purifying the nadis one is able to retain the breath with ease; the gastric fire is increased and experience of (internally aroused) sound and good health are secured.   61

(3:92) By proper practice of pranayama, all diseases are annihilated. Improper practice of pranayama, on the other hand, gives rise to all sorts of diseases.   75

(3:89) Pranayama of a basic level generates sweat, that of an intermediate degree, throbbing. And by pranayama practised in all its intensity, prana raises up (to sushumna). One should perform it in padmasana.   83

4. Pranayama Sadhana

(3:94) One should exhale, retain and inhale in a reg-ulated manner and should in this way attain success in pranayama.   89

(3:91) Just as a lion, an elephant or a tiger is tamed by degrees, similarly respiration is to be brought under control gradually; otherwise it would harm the aspirant.   92

(3:78) After becoming well-versed in asanas, the yogi with his senses under control and eating moderate agreeable food, should practise pranayama as advised by the guru.   109

(3:84) Pranayama should be practised in siddhasana, baddha padmasana or swastikasana, sitting on level ground with the body erect.   110

6. Nadi Shodhana: Purification of the Nadis

(3:82) If the nadis are full of impurities, Maruta (god of wind i.e. prana) does not travel along the middle path (sushumna nadi). How then can one attain the state of unmani? How can one succeed in one's aim?   156

8. Vitalizing Pranayamas

(1:54) Now kapalbhati: Rapid performance of inhalation and exhalation like the bellows of the blacksmith is kapalbhati, well known as the destroyer of all diseases.   199

(1:55) Fast rotation of breathing from left to right and right to left, and exhalation and inhalation is called kapalbhati.   199

10. Pranayama in Spiritual Life

(3:98) One who has mastered pranayama is like Vishnu and Maheshwara. The yogi is like all the gods. Therefore, he should never be disobeyed. 246

PRASHNOPANISHAD

1. Understanding Pranayama

(2:4) In a fit of wrath, prana withdrew himself from the body. Immediately, all the deities found themselves leaving with him, and when prana returned the deities found themselves back in their former places. Just as bees leave the hive when their queen departs and return when she returns, so did the deities behave. Satisfied with this evidence, the deities now give worship to prana. 9

(2:12) O prana, remain in the body calm and quiet; do not leave the body. You are the Lord who abides within the speech, ear, eye and mind. 10

SHIVA SAMHITA

3. Benefits and Effects of Pranayama

(3:40) In the first stage of pranayama, the body of the yogi begins to perspire. When it perspires he should rub it well, otherwise the body of the yogi loses its dhatu (humours). 81

(3:41) In the second stage, there takes place the trembling of the body; in the third, the jumping about like a frog; and when the practice becomes greater, the adept walks in the air. 81

4. Pranayama Sadhana

(3:20) Let the yogi go to a beautiful and pleasant place of retirement or a cell, assume the posture padmasana, and sitting on a seat made of kusha grass, begin to practice the regulation of the breath. 110

(3:31) The following qualities are surely always found in the bodies of every yogi – strong appetite, good digestion, cheerfulness, handsome figure, great courage, mighty enthusiasm and full strength. 112

(3:17) Those who are addicted to sensual pleasures or keep bad company, who are disbelievers, who are devoid of respect towards their guru, who resort to promiscuous assemblies, who are addicted to false and vain controversies, who are cruel in their speech, and who do not give satisfaction to their guru never attain success. 128

(3:18) The first condition of success is the firm belief that it (vidya) must succeed and be fruitful; the second condition is having faith in it; the third is respect towards the guru; the fourth is the spirit of universal equality; the fifth is the restraint of the organs of sense; the sixth is moderate eating, these are all. There is no seventh condition. 130

(3:11) Only the knowledge imparted by a guru, through his lips, is powerful and useful; otherwise it becomes fruitless, weak and painful. 131

6. Nadi Shodhana: Purification of the Nadis

(3:29) The body of the person practising the regulation of breath becomes harmoniously developed, emits sweet scent, and looks beautiful and lovely. 143

(3:22) Then let the wise practitioner close with his right thumb the pingala (right nostril), inspire air through the ida (left nostril) and keep the air confined – suspend the breathing – as long as he can; and afterwards let him breathe out slowly, and not forcibly, through the right nostril. 145

(3:23) Again, let him draw breath through the right nostril, and stop breathing as long as his strength permits; then let him expel the air through the left nostril, not forcibly, but slowly and gently. 145

(3:26) When this (nadi shodhana to 20 counts four times a day) has been practised daily for three months with regularity, the nadis of the body will surely be purified without delay. 152

(3:24) According to the above method of yoga, let him practise twenty kumbhakas (stopping of the breath). He should practise this daily without neglect or idleness, and free from all duals (of love and hatred, and doubt and contention), etc. 153

(3:25) These kumbhakas should be practised four times: once early in the morning at sunrise, then at midday, the third at sunset and the fourth at midnight.   153

10. Pranayama in Spiritual Life

(3:57) When one attains the power of holding the breath for three hours, then certainly the wonderful state of pratyahara is reached without fail.   247

(3:49) The wise practitioner surely destroys all his karma, whether aquired in this life or in the past, through the regulation of the breath.   262

(3:50) The great yogi destroys by sixteen pranayamas the various virtues and vices accumulated in his past life.   262

(3:51) This pranayama destroys sin, as fire burns away a heap of cotton; it makes the yogi free from sin; next it destroys the bonds of all his good actions.   262

(3:52) The mighty yogi, having attained, through pranayama, the eight sorts of psychic powers, and having crossed the ocean of virtue and vice, moves about freely through the three worlds.   264

SRI VIJNANA BHAIRAVA TANTRA

9. Advanced Pranayamas

(25) When the ingoing pranic air and outgoing pranic air are both restrained in their space from their (respective points of) return, the essence of bhairava, which is not different from bhairavi, manifests.   226

(26) When shakti in the form of vayu or pranic air is still and does not move swiftly in a specific direction, there develops in the middle, through the state of nirvikalpa, the form of Bhairava.   227

(27) When kumbhaka takes place after pooraka or rechaka, then the shakti known as shanta is experienced and through that peace (the bhairava consciousness) is revealed.   227

TAITTIRIYA UPANISHAD

1. Understanding Pranayama

Brahmanandavalli (2a): Verily, besides this physical body, which is made of the essence of the food, there is another, inner self comprised of vital energy by which this physical self is filled. Just as the fleshly body is in the form a person, accordingly this vital self is in the shape of a person. 12

YOGA CHUDAMANI UPANISHAD

1. Understanding Pranayama

(v. 89) When the prana moves, the bindu also moves. When the prana remains steady, then the bindu is also steady. Thus the yogi becomes steadfast and firm. Therefore, the prana should be controlled. 17

(v. 92) Even Brahma, fearing a short life span, became a practitioner of pranayama. Therefore, yogis and munis should also control the prana. 26

4. Pranayama Sadhana

(v. 106) Retiring to a solitary place, the yogi should sit in baddha padmasana, with the gaze fixed on the nosetip. Paying homage to the guru, who is Shiva, he should practise pranayama properly. 97

(v. 118) Just as the lion, elephant and tiger are brought under control slowly and steadily, similarly the prana should be controlled, otherwise it becomes destructive to the practitioner. 119

(v. 94) When all the nadis and chakras become free from accumulation of impurities, only then does the yogi becomes capable of controlling the breath. 126

6. Nadi Shodhana: Purification of the Nadis

(v. 101–102) The inhalation, retention and exhalation are the Pranava itself. Pranayama should be practised like this for twelve rounds. Twelve rounds through the ida and pingala nadis unfastens the net of impurities. The yogis should know this always. 140

(v. 99) With full retention of the breath, there is activation of the fire and inner sound is heard. Good health is gained by purification of the nadis. 151

(v. 98) The breath should be drawn in through the left nostril, retained and taken out through the right. Again, the breath should be drawn in through the right and retained, then taken out through the left. By practising this method regularly, one gains control over both points of sun and moon, and the energy channels become purified within two months. 154

7. Tranquillizing Pranayamas

(v. 95) (Sitting) in baddha padmasana, the yogi should inhale the breath through the left nostril, retain it for as long as possible, and exhale again through the right nostril. 180

(v. 96) At the time of pranayama one should meditate on the luminous disc of the moon, which is like the ocean of nectar and white like the milk of cows. 180

8. Vitalizing Pranayamas

(v. 97) At the time of pranayama, the yogi should meditate in the heart on the prescribed zone of the sun, which is blazing brightly. Having established this state, he should be happy. 211

9. Advanced Pranayamas

(v. 100) As long as prana remains in the body, apana should be retained, so that the quantity drawn in one breath remains and moves up and down in hridayakasha. 228

(v. 103) The inhalation should be practised to the count of twelve, retention to the count of sixteen and exhalation to the count of ten. This is called the Omkara pranayama. 229

(v. 104) About pranayama it has been said that the lowest level is twelve counts, the middle level is double that or twenty-four counts, and the highest level is triple or thirty-six counts. 229

(v. 105) The lowest level causes perspiration. The middle level results in trembling of the body. At the highest level stability is achieved. Therefore, the breath should be retained. 231

10. Pranayama in Spiritual Life

(v. 108) In this way, pranayama becomes fire for the fuel of sin, and has always been regarded by the yogis as a great bridge for crossing the ocean of the world.   246

(v. 115) When the prana rises into the sky, inner sounds of musical instruments are produced, like the bell and so on, and the perfection of inner sound is achieved.   251

YOGA SHASTRA OF DATTATREYA

4. Pranayama Sadhana

(v. 107–111) To practise pranayama, the yogi should prepare a small cloister. The door should be small and the room should be free of all germs. The floor and walls should be wiped carefully with cowdung or lime, so that the room remains free of bugs, mosquitoes and spiders. It should be swept daily and perfumed with incense and resin.   129

6. Nadi Shodhana: Purification of the Nadis

(v. 131–132) This (nadi shodhana) should be performed four times a day every day without sloth. This will bring about nadi shuddhi in three months.   143

(v. 178–180) When the unity of prana and apana, manas and prana, and atman and paramatman is attained and their distinctness removed, this stage is called ghatadvayavastha or ghatavastha, for which a regular practice of restraining and sustaining prana is essential. This stage is known by yogis only.   144

(v. 212–215) The stage of parichayavastha comes thereafter if the yogi continues the yoga practice. The prana, acquainted with internal fire, awakens the kundalini and enters without obstacle into the sushumna nadi; the mind also enters into the great path with the prana.   144

YOGA SUTRAS OF SAGE PATANJALI

1. Understanding Pranayama

(2:49) The asana having been done, pranayama is the cessation of the movement of inhalation and exhalation.   19

Glossary

Adhama – lowest, inferior.

Adhara – basis, that which supports, foundation, substratum, receptacle; sixteen specific bases or chakras in the body.

Agni – fire; the god of fire.

Agni tattwa – fire element; fire principle. See Tattwa.

Agnisara kriya – a breathing technique which strengthens the diaphragm and lower stomach region and awakens the digestive fire.

Ajapa – involuntary, unconscious repetition of the same thing, applied especially to the mantra or sound made in breathing, which is 'recited' 21,600 times every 24 hours.

Ajapa japa – continuous, spontaneous repetition of mantra; meditation practice in which mantra is coordinated with breath.

Ajna chakra – psychic/pranic centre situated at the medulla oblongata at the top of the spinal column in the mid-brain; seat of intuition, higher knowledge; third eye.

Akasha tattwa – space element; ether principle. See Tattwa.

Anahad nada – transcendental cosmic sound experienced only in the higher states of meditation; sound which cannot be grasped or heard externally; unproduced or unstruck sound.

Anahata – 'unstruck' or 'unbeaten' sound heard by yogis. See Anahata nada.

Anahata chakra – psychic/pranic centre situated in the spine behind the sternum; associated physically with the cardiac

306

plexus, heart and lungs, mentally with emotion, especially love, and spiritually with atma, the spirit.

Anandamaya kosha – sheath or body of bliss; the innermost wrapper or sheath of the embodied spirit.

Angula – a specific measurement; width of one finger.

Anima siddhi – the power of wilfully making the body small like an atom; the power of making the body subtle. One of the eight major siddhis. See Siddhi.

Annamaya kosha – sheath or body of matter; the sphere of existence created by food, maintained by food and which ultimately becomes food i.e. the body.

Antar – inner.

Antar kumbhaka – internal breath retention; suspension of breath after a full inhalation.

Antar mouna – inner silence; meditative technique belonging to the fifth step of raja yoga (pratyahara).

Antaranga – inner part; internal portion.

Anugraha – divine grace; kindness; assistance.

Apana vayu – one of the pancha pranas or vayus, it is located between the navel and the perineum. It flows downward and controls elimination and reproduction. See Vayu.

Arambha avastha – beginning stage; according to *Hatha Yoga Pradipika* the first state of hearing the inner nada attained after piercing Brahma granthi. See Avastha. See Brahma granthi.

Arjuna – name of the third Pandava brother, who was the son of Lord Indra and Kunti. In the *Bhagavad Gita* he received a divine revelation from Sri Krishna.

Asana – a specific yoga posture; used in hatha yoga to channel prana, open the chakras and remove energy blocks; in raja yoga, a physical posture in which one is at ease and in harmony with oneself.

Ashtanga yoga – the eight limbs of yoga described by Sage Patanjali in the *Yoga Sutras*: yama, niyama, asana, pranayama, pratyahara, dharana, dhyana and samadhi; the ashtanga yoga of Swami Sivananda: serve, love, give, purify, do good, be good, meditate, realize.

Atma – the self beyond mind and body; principle of life, highest reality, Supreme Consciousness, spirit, soul.

Aum – the universal cosmic mantra representing the four states of consciousness; the sound indicating the Supreme Reality or Brahman; conveys concepts of omniscience, omnipresence and omnipotence.

Avastha – state of consciousness or condition of the mind; states of mind in nada yoga practice according to *Hatha Yoga Pradipika*.

Avatara – descent or incarnation of God to the mortal plane.

Ayama – expansion, extension, lengthen; dimension.

Ayurveda – science of health or medicine; the vedic system of medical diagnosis and treatment.

Baddha padmasana – locked lotus pose.

Bahir – external.

Bahir kumbhaka – external breath retention; suspension of breath after a full exhalation.

Bahiranga – external part.

Bandha – psycho-muscular energy locks which close the pranic exits (like throat, anus); psychic locks that concentrate the flow of energy in the body at one point or plexus.

Basti – one of the shatkarmas; yogic enema.

Benares – holy city connected especially with Lord Shiva, also known as Varanasi and Kashi.

Bhagavad Gita – literally, 'divine song'; Sri Krishna's discourse to his disciple Arjuna delivered on the battlefield of Kurukshetra at the commencement of the great Mahabharata war; one of the source books of Hindu philosophy, containing the essence of the Upanishads and yoga.

Bhairava – the name of Lord Shiva in his fierce aspect; state of consciousness which preceds the ultimate experience of universal consciousness or Shiva.

Bhairavi – Bhairavi is Shiva's consort or Shakti, i.e. the power that manifests this particular aspect of existence. See Bhairava.

Bhoomi tyaga – a yogic accomplishment where the body becomes so light that it is able to leave or rise above the earth.

Bhrumadhya – trigger point for ajna chakra located at the eyebrow centre.

Bhu samadhi – yogic state achieved through prolonged kumbhaka where all vital functions appear to have ceased and the yogi is buried in the earth.

Bija mantra – seed sound; a basic mantra or syllable.

Bindu – point; seed, source, drop; point of potential energy and consciousness, used in kriya yoga; the basis from which emanated the first principle according to the tantra shastra; nucleus; psychic centre located in the brain; in tantra and hatha yoga it also represents a drop of semen.

Brahma – god of the Hindu trinity who creates the universe; God as creator; manifest force of life and creation; ever-expanding, limitless consciousness; Absolute Reality.

Brahma granthi – psychic/muscular 'knot' of creation, situated in mooladhara chakra, symbolizing material and sensual attachment. See Granthi.

Brahmacharya – being absorbed in higher consciousness; sublimation of sexual energy for spiritual development; celibacy; conduct suitable for proceeding to the highest state of existence; one of the five yamas described by Sage Patanjali in the *Yoga Sutras* as a preliminary practice of yoga.

Brahmamuhurta – the two hours around sunrise (in India between 4 am and 6 am) best suited to yoga sadhana.

Brahman – etymologically 'ever expanding, limitless consciousness'; name of Supreme Consciousness or cosmic intelligence according to Vedanta philosophy; God as creator; monistic concept of Absolute Reality.

Brahmarandhra – crown of the head; the fontanelle; opening in the crown of the head through which the soul is said to escape on leaving the body.

Buddhi – discerning, discriminating aspect of the mind; aspect of the mind closest to pure consciousness; one of the four parts of the antahkarana or inner instrument.

Chakra – circle, wheel or vortex; pranic/psychic centre; confluence point of energy flows (nadis) in the body; the seven major chakras for descent of divine energy or for human evolution are sahasrara, ajna, vishuddhi, anahata, manipura, swadhisthana and mooladhara.

Chandra – moon; representing the mental energy. See Ida nadi.

Chidakasha – the space of consciousness; the inner space visualized in meditation behind the closed eyes or in the region of ajna chakra.

Chin mudra – psychic gesture of consciousness; a hand mudra. See Mudra.

Chitta – individual consciousness, including the subconscious and unconscious layers of mind; thinking, concentration, attention, enquiry; storehouse of memory or samskaras; one of the four parts of the antahkarana or inner instrument.

Chitta shakti – the power of pure consciousness; mental force governing the subtle dimensions.

Chitta shuddhi – purification of the mind; purity of consciousness.

Danda – a yoga danda is a u-shaped wooden prop that is placed under the armpit, regulating the breath by its pressure, used by yogis in sadhana; 'danda' means stick or symbol of authority or discipline.

Danda kriya – the act of resting the armpit on a danda, a stick, to influence the swara (flow of breath in the nostrils).

Dattatreya, Sage – an ancient sage who learned from twenty-four gurus; considered to be an incarnation of Brahma, Vishnu and Shiva; author of *Yoga Shastra of Dattatreya*.

Deva – being of light; divine being.

Devi – female deity, goddess.

Dharana – practice of concentration or complete attention; sixth stage of ashtanga yoga described in Sage Patanjali's *Yoga Sutras* as holding or binding the mind to one point.

Dhatu – seven constituents of the body: blood, bone, marrow, fat, semen, skin and flesh.

Dhauti – one of the shatkarmas; cleansing techniques for the digestive system, chest and head.

Dhyana – spontaneous state of meditation; one-pointedness of mind through concentration on either a form, thought or sound; absorption in the object of meditation; seventh stage of Sage Patanjali's ashtanga yoga.

Dosha – three humours of the body described in Ayurveda: mucus (kapha), bile (pitta) and wind (vata). Their imbalance prevents the flow of energy in sushumna nadi.

Ganga – the river Ganges, the most sacred river in India; pingala nadi.

Garima siddhi – the power of making the body heavy at will. One of the eight major siddhis. See Siddhi.

Gayatri mantra – a most sacred twenty-four syllable mantra which enables learning.

Ghata avastha – the second state of hearing the inner nada according to *Hatha Yoga Pradipika*; state of nada attained when shakti enters the chitrini nadi within sushumna.

Gheranda Samhita – traditional text on hatha yoga by Sage Gheranda. It explains seven limbs (saptanga) of yoga: shatkarma, asana, mudra, pratyahara, pranayama, dhyana and samadhi.

Gheranda, Sage – author of *Gheranda Samhita*, a classical yoga text which describes seven limbs of yoga.

Granthi – psychic knot; the three granthis on the sushumna nadi which hinder the upward passage of kundalini, viz. Brahma granthi, Vishnu granthi and Rudra granthi. See Brahma granthi. See Rudra granthi. See Vishnu granthi.

Guna – quality; the three gunas, qualities or aspects of prakriti/nature are sattwa, rajas and tamas.

Guru – one who dispels the darkness caused by ignorance (avidya); teacher of the science of ultimate reality who by the light of his own atma can dispel darkness, ignorance and illusion from the mind and enlighten the consciousness of a devotee/disciple; preceptor.

Ha – seed mantra of solar energy, pranic force (pingala nadi); represents sun; first syllable of the word 'hatha'. See Tha.

311

Ham – mantra produced by the breath, unconsciously repeated on exhalation; representing individual consciousness; bija mantra of the space element and vishuddhi chakra. See So. See Soham.

Hamso – mantra used in ajapa japa; correlate of the mantra Soham. See Soham.

Hasta – hand.

Hatha yoga – a system of yoga specifically using practices for bodily purification; yoga of attaining physical and mental purity and balancing the prana (energy) in ida and pingala nadis so that sushumna nadi opens, enabling the experiences of samadhi. See Ha. See Tha.

Hatha Yoga Pradipika – a major classical text on hatha yoga compiled by Yogi Swatmarama, usually translated as 'light on hatha yoga'.

Hatharatnavali – a late medieval treatise on hatha yoga and tantra by Srinivasa Bhatta Mahayogindra.

Hridayakasha – psychic space of the heart centre where the creative hues of emotion are observed; experienced between manipura and vishuddhi chakras, associated with anahata chakra.

Ida nadi – a major pranic channel running from the left side of mooladhara chakra to the left side of ajna chakra, governing the left side of the body and the right side of the brain. The ida energy flow criss-crosses the spine through the major chakras between mooladhara and ajna, conducting the passive aspect of prana manifesting as the mental force, lunar force or chitta shakti; also called chandra nadi as the lunar energy flows through it.

Indriya – sense organ; power of the senses; power.

Ishitva siddhi – the power to wilfully create and destroy. One of the eight major siddhis. See Siddhi.

Jagrat – the waking state; dimension of consciousness, related to the senses and the phenomenal material universe.

Jala tattwa – water element, water principle. See Tattwa.

Jalandhara bandha – throat lock; practice in which the chin rests forward upon the upper sternum.

Japa – a meditation practice involving repetition of a mantra.

Jiva – principle of life; individual or personal soul; living being.

Jivatma – individual or personal soul.

Jnana – knowledge, cognition, wisdom; higher knowledge derived from meditation or from inner experience.

Jnanendriya – organ of sense perceptions and knowledge; five in number, viz. ears, eyes, nose, tongue and skin.

Jyoti – a small flame; light, brightness; fire.

Kabir Das – (1440–1518) a poet and mystic, his teachings blend Hinduism, Sufism and bhakti.

Kaivalya – final liberation; highest state of samadhi; that state of consciousness which is beyond duality.

Kali Yuga – the present age, last of the four ages or cycles in the Day of Brahma and Maha Yuga, which began in 3,102 BC and has a duration of 432,000 years. During this cycle man is collectively at the height of technology, decadence, dishonesty and corruption of spiritual awareness; dark, evil, difficult and full of strife.

Kamadeva – the god of love.

Kapalbhati – frontal brain cleansing breath; one of the six major cleansing techniques, shatkarmas of hatha yoga; process of purifying the frontal region of the brain by breathing rapidly through the nostrils with emphasis on exhalation.

Kapha – mucus, phlegm, one of the three humours (doshas) described in Ayurveda; associated with the water element. See Dosha.

Karma – action and result; law of cause and effect.

Karmendriya – motor organ; there are five physical organs of action, viz. vocal cords, hands, feet, genital organ and anus.

Kevala kumbhaka – spontaneous retention of breath.

Khechari mudra – literally, 'the attitude of moving in space'; tongue lock; a hatha yoga practice in which the elongated tongue passes back into the pharynx to stimulate the flow of life-giving nectar (amrita), whereas in the milder raja yoga form the tongue is inserted in, or folded backwards towards, the upper cavity of the palate.

Kosha – sheath or body; a dimension of experience and existence. The five koshas are: annamaya kosha, pranamaya kosha, manomaya kosha, vijnanamaya kosha, and anandamaya kosha.

Krishna, Sri – literally, 'black' or 'dark'; eighth incarnation of Vishnu; avatara who descended in the Dwapara Yuga. Sri Krishna is perhaps the most celebrated hero in Hindu mythology and seems to be an historical figure. To uphold dharma he orchestrated the Mahabharata war. His teachings to his friend and disciple Arjuna during that war are immortalized in the *Bhagavad Gita*.

Kriya – action; cleansing practice (shatkarma); practice of kriya yoga.

Kriya yoga – practices of kundalini yoga designed to speed the evolution of humanity.

Kumbhaka – internal or external retention of the breath.

Kundalini – the evolutionary energy in a human being; spiritual energy; Devi described as the potential energy of a human being dormant in mooladhara chakra, which, when awakened, awakens the chakras, resulting in progressive enlightenment.

Kundalini yoga – path of yoga which awakens the dormant spiritual force, kundalini. See Kundalini.

Kunjal – cleansing the stomach by voluntary vomiting using warm saline water; one of the hatha yoga shatkarmas (cleansing techniques).

Kurma nadi – a pranic channel in the throat.

Laghima siddhi – the power of wilfully making the body light. One of the eight major siddhis. See Siddhi.

Laghoo shankhaprakshalana – short intestinal wash; a practice of dhauti; one of the hatha yoga shatkarmas (cleansing techniques).

Laya yoga – literally, 'union by absorption'; yoga of conscious dissolution of individuality.

314

Madhyama – medium, intermediate; intermediate sound, the second stage of nada yoga; also called whispering sound (upanshu). See Nada yoga.

Maha bandha – the great lock; a combination of jalandhara bandha, uddiyana bandha and moola bandha, practised with external breath retention.

Mahaprana – cosmic, universal prana.

Mahatma – literally, 'great soul'; used with reference to a person who has destroyed the ego and realized the self as one with all.

Maheshwara – great lord, sovereign; name of Shiva. See Ishwara.

Mahima siddhi – the power of wilfully making the body large. One of the eight major siddhis. See Siddhi.

Makarasana – crocodile pose; a relaxation posture with backward bend.

Manas – finite mind, rational mind; the mind concerned with senses, thought and counter-thought; perception, intelligence; one of the four parts of the antahkarana or inner instrument.

Manas shakti – mental energy.

Manas tattwa – element representing the mind.

Manipura chakra – literally, 'city of jewels'; psychic/pranic centre situated in the spine behind the navel; associated with the solar plexus and digestive organs and mentally with willpower; source of vitality and energy.

Manolaya – involution and dissolution of the mind unto its cause.

Manomaya kosha – mental sheath or body; mental sphere of life and awareness.

Mantra – words of power; sound vibrations which liberate the mind when repeated.

Manu – the first law-giver, father of the human race.

Marga – path.

Maruta – another word for prana; god of wind.

Matra – unit of time; time interval in pronouncing a vowel; standard measure, rule; unit.

Maya – means by which Brahman creates the phenomenal world; power of creation; illusive power; in Vedanta philosophy, the two powers of maya are: 1. the power of veiling, and 2. the power of projection; in Samkhya philosophy, another name for Prakriti.

Mitahara – sattwic food; fresh and digestible food eaten moderately and appreciatively.

Moola bandha – perineum contraction; contraction of the perineal body in the male and the cervix in the female body; technique used for locating and awakening mooladhara chakra.

Mooladhara chakra – the lowest psychic/pranic centre in the human body; situated in the perineal floor in men and the cervix in women; associated physically with the coccygeal plexus, excretory and reproductive organs, and mentally with the instinctive nature; spiritually it is the seat of kundalini.

Mudra – gesture; psychic, emotional, devotional, and aesthetic gestures; attitudes of energy intended to link individual pranic force with universal or cosmic force; grain, as one of the panchamakara of tantra.

Mukhya – chief, principal, foremost, prominent.

Muni – one who contemplates; one who has conquered the mind; one who maintains silence or stillness of mind.

Nada – sound; subtle sound or vibration created by the union of the Shiva and Shakti tattwas; the first manifestation of the unmanifest Absolute.

Nada yoga – the process of penetrating deeper and deeper into the nature of one's own reality by listening to subtle inner sounds.

Nadi – flow; a river or channel of energy; psychic current; subtle channel in the pranic body, conducting the flow of shakti; comparable to the meridians of acupuncture.

Nadi shuddhi – cleansing of the pathways of prana, nadis.

Nasikagra – tip of the nose.

Nasikagra drishti – nosetip gazing; a practice to stimulate mooladhara chakra.

Nauli – abdominal massaging; one of the shatkarmas in which the rectus abdominis muscles are contracted and isolated vertically.

Neti – one of the shatkarmas; nasal cleansing with saline water (jala neti), a waxed string (sutra neti) or other elements.

Nigraha – control.

Nirgarbha – without repetition of mantra. See Sagarbha.

Nirvana – cessation of suffering; final liberation or emancipation in Buddhist thought.

Nirvikalpa samadhi – state in which the mind ceases to function and only pure consciousness remains; superconscious state where mental modifications cease to exist, resulting in transcendence of the manifest world.

Nishpatti avastha – fourth and final state of hearing the inner nada according to *Hatha Yoga Pradipika,* equated with nirvikalpa samadhi which renders one a jivanmukta.

Niyama – observance of rules or rules of personal discipline to render the mind tranquil in preparation for meditation; the second step of the eight limbs (ashtanga yoga) of Sage Patanjali in the *Yoga Sutras*: shaucha (purity), santosha (contentment), tapas (austerity), swadhyaya (self-study) and Ishwara pranidhana (surrender to God).

Om – See Aum.

Padadhirasana – breath balancing pose.

Padmasana – lotus pose; classical meditative posture.

Pancha dharana – five kinds of concentration on the five elements.

Pancha prana – five major divisions of the pranic energy located in the physical body, viz. apana, prana, samana, udana, vyana; also called vayu.

Paramatma – cosmic Soul or Consciousness; Supreme Self; the atma of the entire universe; God.

Parananda – transcendental bliss; higher state of awareness.

Parichaya avastha – state of increase, the third state of nada yoga according to *Hatha Yoga Pradipika*.

Patanjali, Sage – author of the *Yoga Sutras*; an ancient rishi who codified the system of raja yoga, including ashtanga yoga.

Pingala nadi – a major pranic channel in the body which conducts the dynamic pranic force manifesting as prana shakti from the right side of mooladhara chakra, criss-crossing the spine through the major chakras to the right side of ajna chakra; associated with the mundane realm of experience and externalized awareness; also called surya nadi as the solar energy flows through it.

Pitta – bile, one of the three humours (doshas) described in Ayurveda; associated with the fire element. See Dosha.

Pooraka – the first stage of pranayama; breathing in.

Prakamya siddhi – the power of unobstructed fulfilment of desire. One of the eight major siddhis. See Siddhi.

Prakash – light, brightness, shining, brilliance.

Prana – vital energy force sustaining life and creation, permeating the whole of creation and existing in both the macrocosmos and microcosmos.

Prana nigraha – control of breath; preliminary practices of breath regulation and control before proper pranayama begins. See Pranayama.

Prana shakti – energy; dynamic solar force governing the dimension of matter; energy flow related to externalization of mind; the force of prana.

Prana tattwa – element representing the vital or life-giving force.

Prana vayu – pranic air current; also refers to a specific current, one of the pancha pranas or vayus, located in the thoracic region, from the throat to the diaphragm, responsible for processes of inspiration and absorption.

Prana vidya – knowledge and control of prana; a healing technique involving awareness and movement of prana.

Pranamaya kosha – energy sheath, or vital pranic body; the sheath covering the self which is composed of pranic vibration and the rhythm of pranic forces.

Pranava – another word for the sacred syllable *Aum* or *Om*, the primal sound vibration, the symbol of the Soul or Self.

Pranavadin – a hatha yogi; one who lives according to the pranic sciences.

318

Pranayama – a series of techniques using the breath to control the flow of prana within the body.

Pranotthana – awakening of the pranas in the different nadis and chakras; a stage of awakening preparatory to kundalini awakening.

Prapti siddhi – the power of acquiring everything. One of the eight major siddhis. See Siddhi.

Prashnopanishad – name of an Upanishad consisting of six questions and the corresponding answers given by Sage Pippalada after the seekers had served in his ashram for one year.

Pratyahara – restraining the sensory and motor organs; withdrawal and emancipation of the mind from the domination of the senses and sensual objects; training the senses to follow the mind within; fifth stage of ashtanga yoga described by Sage Patanjali in the *Yoga Sutras*.

Prithvi tattwa – earth element, earth principle. See Tattwa.

Purushartha – human attainment; self-effort; the four basic needs or desires to be fulfilled in life, viz. artha (wealth), kama (desire), dharma (duty), moksha (liberation).

Raja – king, chief.

Raja yoga – the supreme yoga; union through control of the mental processes and concentration of the mind; the most authoritative text is Sage Patanjali's *Yoga Sutras* which contains ashtanga yoga, the eightfold path.

Rajas – one of the three gunas or attributes of nature; dynamism; state of activity; creativity combined with full ego involvement. See Guna.

Rama, Sri – the seventh avatara of Vishnu and embodiment of dharma, hero of the epic *Ramayana*; a heroic and virtuous king.

Ramana Maharshi – (1879–1950) a renowned jnana yogi and enlightened sage who taught mainly through silence; establisher of the path of self-enquiry.

Rechaka – the process of exhalation in pranayama; emptying of the lungs.

Rishi – seer; realized sage; one who contemplates or meditates on the Self.

Roopa – form; appearance.

Rudra granthi – literally, 'knot of Rudra (Shiva)'; psychic knot within ajna chakra which symbolizes attachment to siddhis or higher mental attributes. As the psychic block is overcome, the sense of personal identity ceases to block one's identification with the cosmic consciousness. See Granthi.

Sadhaka – one who practises sadhana; a spiritual aspirant.

Sadhana – spiritual practice or discipline performed regularly.

Sadhu – holy person, sage, saint.; renunciate

Sagarbha – impregnated; with repetition of mantra. See Nirgarbha.

Sahita – combined with something; accompanied, attended by, together with.

Sahita kumbhaka – pranayama in which inhalation, retention and exhalation are practised.

Sakshi – that which observes the phenomenal reality without being affected at all; witness.

Samadhi – the culmination of meditation, state of oneness of the mind with the object of concentration and the universal consciousness; self-realization; the eighth stage of raja yoga.

Samana vayu – one of the five pancha pranas or vayus, it is located between the navel and the diaphragm; it flows from side to side and controls the digestion. See Vayu.

Samskara – mental impression stored in the subtle body as an archetype; the impressions which condition one's nature, causing one to react or respond in a certain way.

Sandhya – three times of day when there is a confluence of energies – sunrise, noon and sunset; transition; union; division.

Sannyasa – dedication; complete renunciation of the world, its possessions and attachments; abandonment of the phenomenal world.

Sannyasin – one who has taken sannyasa initiation, surrendering everything to the guru and the spiritual journey.

Sapta dhatu – the seven dhatus. See Dhatu.

Sattwa – one of the three gunas, or attributes of nature; state of luminosity, harmony, equilibrium and purity. See Guna.

Shabda – sound; perceptible sound; object of the sense of hearing and property of space; word.

Shakti – primal energy; manifest consciousness; power, ability, capacity, strength, energy; counterpart of Shiva; the moving power of nature and consciousness; in Hindu mythology Shakti is often symbolized as a divine woman.

Shambhavi mudra – eyebrow centre gazing; psychic attitude focused on Shiva (Supreme Consciousness).

Shankhaprakshalana – literally, 'cleaning the conch'; a cleansing technique (shatkarma) of hatha yoga that uses saline water to clean the stomach (which is shaped like a conch) and the small and large intestines.

Sharada – autumn.

Sharira – the body (of animate or inanimate objects).

Shashankasana – the hare pose; a forward bending asana performed from vajrasana.

Shatkarma – the six hatha yoga techniques of purification: neti, dhauti, basti, nauli, kapalbhati and trataka.

Shavasana – the corpse pose; a relaxation posture.

Shiva – state of pure consciousness, individual and cosmic, original source of yoga. Lord of yogis; auspicious, benevolent one; name of the god of the Hindu trinity who is entrusted with the work of destruction; destroyer of the ego and duality.

Shiva Samhita – Sanskrit text enumerating the concepts and principles essential to the practice of yoga; classical text on hatha yoga.

Shodhana – first limb of Sage Gheranda's saptanga yoga; purification.

Shoonya – void, state of transcendental consciousness; space behind the eyebrow centre.

Shvasa – breath.

Siddha yoni asana – classical meditation posture, the male equivalent is siddhasana.

Siddhasana – accomplished pose; classical cross-legged meditation posture.

Siddhi – perfection; enhanced pranic and psychic capacity; paranormal or supernormal accomplishment; control of mind and prana; eight supernatural powers obtained by yogis as a result of long practice.

So – mantra produced by the breath, unconsciously repeated on inhalation; representing cosmic consciousness. See Ham. See Soham.

Soham – mantra used in ajapa japa, said to be the unconscious repetitive prayer produced by the breath itself.

Sri Yantra – geometric diagram representing the divine 'female' energy, or shakti.

Sthoola – gross.

Sukhasana – easy pose; a cross-legged meditation asana.

Sukra nadi – a pranic channel in the perineum, the area between the excretory and urinary organs.

Sukshma – subtle; relating to the world of the psyche.

Surya nadi – literally 'energy flow of the sun'; another name for pingala nadi. See Pingala nadi.

Sushumna – central energy flow (nadi) in the spine; it conducts the kundalini or spiritual force from mooladhara chakra to sahasrara chakra; the main energy flow related to transcendental awareness; situated in the spinal cord of the human body, it opens when balance is achieved between ida and pingala nadis.

Sushupti – third dimension of consciousness; deep sleep or unconscious realm of mind; profound repose undisturbed by the senses.

Sutra – thread; condensed statements strung together to give an outline of a philosophy, such as the *Yoga Sutras* of Sage Patanjali.

Swadhisthana chakra – literally, 'one's own abode'; second psychic/pranic centre; located in the coccyx; associated with the sacral plexus and governing the urogenital system; the storehouse of subconscious impressions.

Swami – literally, 'master of the mind'; master of the self; title of sannyasins.

Swapna – second dimension of consciousness; subconscious realm of mind, state of dreaming, the mind is looking inwards, seeing the internal experience, not the external objects.

Swara – breathing cycle; flow of the breath in the nostrils.

Swara yoga – science of the breathing cycle; the system of yoga using understanding and management of the breathing cycle as a means to attain self-realization.

Swastikasana – auspicious pose; a cross-legged meditation asana.

Swatmarama, Yogi – literally, 'one who revels within oneself'; the author of *Hatha Yoga Pradipika*, a classical text book on hatha yoga.

Tamas – one of the three gunas or attributes of nature; inertia, stability; ignorance, darkness; unwillingness to change. See Guna.

Tantra – a most ancient universal science and culture which deals with the transition of human nature from the present level of evolution and understanding to a transcendental level of knowledge, experience and awareness; a particular path of sadhana including mantra, yantra and other esoteric practices.

Tapa – heat.

Tapas – austerity; undergoing hardship for the purpose of purification; pain of three types: *adhyatmika*, spiritual, *adhidevika*, natural or environmental, and *adhibhautika*, physical; one of the niyamas described by Sage Patanjali in the *Yoga Sutras* as a preliminary practice of yoga. See Niyama.

Tattwa – 'that-ness'; true essential nature; an element, a primary substance; the five elements (space, air, fire, water and earth); another name for mahabhoota.

Tha – seed mantra of lunar energy, psychic or mental force (ida nadi); represents moon; second syllable of the word 'hatha'. See Ha.

Trataka – one of the shatkarmas; a technique of gazing steadfastly upon an object such as a candle flame, black dot or yantra with unblinking eyes.

Tulsidas – author of one of the versions of the famous epic *Ramayana* called the *Ramacharitamanas*, which describes the life of Sri Rama. It is composed in poetic form and is chanted by devotees throughout India.

Turiya – fourth dimension of consciousness; superconsciousness; simultaneous awareness of the conscious, subconscious and unconscious mind which links and transcends them; a state of liberation.

Udana vayu – one of the five pancha pranas or vayus, it is located in the extremities of the body: arms, legs and head; it flows with a spiralling motion and rises up the throat entering the head; it controls the sensory and motor organs. See Vayu.

Uddiyana bandha – abdominal retraction lock; drawing in of the abdomen towards the backbone after exhaling.

Unmani – mindless; beyond the mind.

Uttama – highest, best; principal.

Vairagya – non-attachment; absence of sensual craving and desires; detachment; supreme dispassion.

Vajrasana – thunderbolt pose; a kneeling meditative posture.

Vasanta – the season of spring.

Vashitva siddhi – the power of gaining control over everything. One of the eight major siddhis. See Siddhi.

Vasishtha, Sage – a celebrated rishi and seer of the Vedas; guru of Sri Rama; author of many vedic hymns. His teachings are recorded in *Yoga Vasishtha*, one of the greatest expositions of jnana yoga.

Vata – wind, gas; one of the three humours (doshas) described in Ayurveda; associated with the air element. See Dosha.

Vatsara dhauti – a technique of dhauti, one of the six cleansing practices of hatha yoga (shatkarma), in which air is swallowed into the stomach and belched out.

Vayu – god of wind; wind, air; life breath or vital air, used as another name for prana, of which there are five main types, viz. prana, apana, samana, udana and vyana, also called pancha prana.

Vidya – knowledge or science, particularly knowledge of spiritual truth and non-mundane reality.

Vijnana Bhairava Tantra – a text on branches of tantra, particularly the yogachara path of practice.

Vishnu – vedic deity; the second deity of the Hindu trinity (Brahma, Vishnu, Shiva), entrusted with the preservation of the universe, a duty which obliges him to appear in several incarnations; Supreme Consciousness.

Vishnu granthi – psychic block or knot particularly related to manipura, anahata and vishuddhi chakras, symbolizing the bondage of personal and emotional attachment. See Granthi.

Vishuddhi chakra – literally, 'centre of purification', the psychic/pranic centre located at the level of the throat pit or the thyroid gland; it is the psychic centre particularly connected with purification and communication.

Viveka buddhi – discriminative intellect.

Vritti – a modification arising in the mind related to a thought pattern; a particular mental state or condition.

Vyana vayu – one of the pancha pranas or vayus; the reserve of pranic energy pervading the entire body. See Vayu.

Yama – self-restraints or rules of conduct which render the mind tranquil; first stage of the eight limbs of yoga (ashtanga yoga) of Sage Patanjali's *Yoga Sutras*: ahimsa (non-violence), satya (truth), asteya (honesty), brahmacharya (continence) and aparigraha (abstention from greed).

Yami – one who practices control or restraint.

Yoga – union; the root is yuj, meaning 'to join', 'to yoke'; a system of practice leading to a state of union between the individual and universal awareness; practices, philosophy and lifestyle to achieve peace, power and spiritual wisdom as well as perfect health, a sound mind and a balanced personality; one of the six main systems of Indian philosophy.

Yoga Chudamani Upanishad – a yogic text elucidating a unique combination of kundalini yoga and vedantic upasana.

Yoga nidra – psychic sleep; practice in which the body sleeps while the mind remains aware as its movements are guided and quietened by instructions, inducing deep relaxation of body, mind and emotions.

Yoga Shastras – the yoga system of philosophy and practice where the chief aim is to teach the means for the human soul to unite completely with the Supreme Spirit; elaborate rules for the proper practice of concentration of mind.

Yoga Sutras – ancient authoritative text on raja yoga by Sage Patanjali.

Yoga Taravali – a poetic summary of the highest teachings of yoga by Adi Shankaracharya, the founder of Advaita Vedanta.

Yoga Upanishads – a group of approximately twenty-two Upanishads more specifically concerned with yoga.

Yoga Vasishtha – a monumental scripture on Vedanta in the form of a dialogue between Sri Rama and his guru Sage Vasishtha.

Yogi, yogin – an adept of yoga; follower of the yoga system of philosophy and practice.

Yogini – a female adept of yoga; female follower of the yoga system of philosophy and practice.

Yukta, yuktam – literally 'one who is in a state of yoga'; union; precision; appropriateness.

General Index